I See You

I See You

Published by Bell Asteri Publishing & Enterprises, LLC
209 West 2nd Street #177
Fort Worth TX 76102
www.bellasteri.com

Published in the United States of America

ISBN: 978-1-957604-16-9 (hardback)
ISBN: 978-1-957604-17-6 (paperback)
ISBN: 978-1-957604-19-0 (electronic book)

Introduction

Shari Ann Almeida was a wife, mother and career woman before she became a cancer mom. Writing was something she did after cheering at a Friday night football game, incognito in the corner of a bookstore. It wasn't until her six-month old baby Dakota was diagnosed with cancer that the world saw her hidden words. Writing it all down was a way of giving validation to the feelings that had no words. She chose to put her story out there on stage in the spotlight. But she didn't do it for her or her family. It was for the people like them. She just didn't know it yet.

This story gives a brutally honest look into the cruelty of pediatric cancer, and takes the reader on a journey filled with anguish and pain. Her writing style is very poetic and beautiful, yet fiercely troublesome for how could it not be? Babies fighting cancer is the epitome of troublesome. "I See You" is the first in a series of books that are written to remind all of the cancer parents out there that they are not alone. They may feel isolated, but they are seen.

CHAPTER 1

*I*t had been 41 days since I had last taken a pregnancy test. I didn't smile or jump for joy. I didn't run out to the store at four in the morning to buy onesies and gift bags. Instead, I held my belly like a basket cradles eggs, praying it wasn't empty. I sat on the couch and waited for him to wake up. When I told him, he didn't pick me up and spin me around like the last time. His face matched my own and I have no doubt his stomach was in his throat too. The test results came in right before my big interview, giving me a boost of hope. On a Friday afternoon, we drove to our first ultrasound while throwing confetti into the wind celebrating my new job opportunity. We must have overspent our happiness vouchers because they couldn't find a heartbeat. We held one another on the edge of the table, sobbing at what we thought would be our greatest heartbreak.

The drive home was the complete opposite of the drive there. No more talk of names, colors or *to-dos*. We barely caught one another's gaze out of fear that we'd break or worse, we would fail one another. I had a slip in my hand that was meant to help ease the situation. Just the presence of the paper infuriated him and only made the car go faster. At home we discussed options while making every attempt to not drown. My husband being the "demand for answers" type, requested a second opinion. Me being the "failure at heart" kind, didn't want to face my body losing again. Monday morning, I made the call to have another ultrasound. I was scheduled for Thursday morning to confirm and Friday morning to complete the incomplete pregnancy.

Thursday, at 9:30 a.m., there was still no heartbeat. I was asked to come back at 3:30 to confirm one final time. I went to the bookstore, coffee in hand, and lost myself amongst the minds of others. I was desperate to be anywhere but here, so I used their words as jet plane tickets to help pass the time. By 3:00, I was in the car, sweaty palms leading the way, screaming at the sky pretending someone could hear my voice. Lying on the table, I wouldn't even look at the monitor as it would make this nightmare all the more real. She asked me to look, and I felt as if she had asked me to willingly drink bleach. She asked again, and fighting every millimeter of my head turn, I looked. It was love at first sight, the first time I saw my baby.

The room was swimming in tears and our bleeding hearts were our lifejackets. We more or less skipped down the hall to the original place of terror where they, too, were floating on waves of pure happiness. The universe had decided we still had two pennies to rub together and we were not going to waste one cent. I protected the flower growing in my belly with my every breath. I was mindful of every speck of air around me and each piece that went down the hatch. Barely lapping mile five, bound and determined to finish strong beyond mile nine.

Because my husband and I are both type A and OCD, we couldn't wait to know the gender, so we found out at 16 weeks. We knew we had created this baby as its legs were crossed the entire time, forcing me to roll around like a dog in a mud puddle in attempts to find an answer. In our hearts, we already knew there was only one gender who could make us work this hard for a sliver of information. Giggling up a storm I am sure, there she was, our Dakota Ann. Terrified and overjoyed, all in the same breath, as I am all to aware of the sugar and spice. I had always loathed the color pink, ruffles, glitter - all of the things that defined girls. I have a romance with the color black, push-ups and squats - everything that is the opposite of femininity. As I mentioned before, the universe likes to keep me in check more often than I care to admit.

I spent my pregnancy finding all of the prettiest blues, avoiding every shade of pink, running hills with her motivation, and preparing for the more than prepared. She came into this world with a mermaid thumb and a strawberry blonde cowlick to boot. Her blue eyes held captive my stare, as if to say, "Oh there you are." She fed from me immediately and this was the easiest mountain we'd climb. We were drunk in baby love and a level of exhausted we assumed had no other elevations. She was rolling over at three weeks old, standing by two months old and we needed freezers for our freezers full of breastmilk. I upheld my promise to myself to be a mom, a wife and a career woman, although leaving her was like severing my arm from my shoulder every time. I helicoptered my mom on the hour every hour being sure to be overly present even when I wasn't present. There are too many books on how to parent too far to the right, and I was acing every test in my naïve pompous opinion, until I failed catastrophically.

She preferred howling at the moon over sleep and hated to be alone. One night while she was practicing her wolf song in her crib, I reached down to pick her up and she was soaked as if she had been submerged in a pool. I changed her navy blue onesie with the bear on it and noticed that her diaper was dry. With my forehead birthing folds and my lips pursed, I put the mishap in my "weird box" and moved along as if I had moments to spare. There was another early morning similar to this event, but there had been weeks in between. So, I put another check in the "strange column" and strolled all too quickly into the next task up ahead. She had begun teething by three months old which sparked on-again off-again low-grade fevers, accompanied by a runny nose. I gave her Tylenol when she seemed too uncomfortable, hoping to instill grit, and focused on her medals to be obtained while pounding into a spring floor. She had some faint, pale green bruising along the right side of her body (small in size), on her thigh, ribcage, tricep and cheek. There were tiny purple dots on the bottom of her left buttock which threw me for loop. I placed yet another check mark in the "off column" and pressed play while being tempted to hit fast forward. Then the universe hit pause. Every piece laid out above, from here on out, will be forever known as our *before*.

Wednesday, April 24, 2019 is Day One of life as we cannot unknow it. At her six months well visit, her pediatrician decided not to administer any vaccinations due to her low-grade fever. She mentioned the marks on her body I had blatantly bulldozed and the look on her face told me my character was possibly in question. I assured her that my touch would never harm Dakota's body and in the awkward moment, she sent us for bloodwork. I was doused in gasoline and lit ablaze, screaming obscenities to the sunny skies. I thought helping two other people hold her down for bloodwork that afternoon was a horror scene from hell. At home on our couch, at 3:00 p.m., my phone alerted me with preliminary results reading within normal limits. With normal results, we went about our normal day and I fed her self-pureed pears. Within the hour, my phone rang - the phone call that changed our lives for forever. Her pediatrician said, "I need you to get Dakota to the nearest emergency room with a pediatric hematologist. There is something wrong with Dakota's blood." I frantically packed her diaper bag with not enough diapers or clothes and a bag of milk. With a watermelon growing in the back of my throat, we left our home, not knowing we'd never come back.

My options were a local hospital less than 40 minutes away or a bigger hospital well over an hour away. I drove for less than 30 minutes. I threw a blanket over her, walking through the ER parking lot as if I could shield her from the demons that were already raging a war inside her. Dakota's Pop Pop walked behind us, assuring us that everything was okay, but I knew in my bones that nothing was okay. Those automatic doors closed behind us, symbolizing the end of everything we had known and the beginning of a treacherous new. Within seconds, we were in an isolated room, her in my lap adorned with wires like an octopus with 20 extra tentacles. Another room, with far too many people, more wiring limiting my access to her skin that hours ago was just beneath my fingertips. Forget howling at the moon. She was beckoning every unseen power to fix the situation and I was pleading to the universe right alongside her.

The room was spinning with unanswered questions. Our vision was intoxicated from losing our grip inside the funnel. I climbed onto the bed with her between my legs. We were wheeled through hallways like morning woods during the first snow, so cold I swear I could see our breath. That hell scene of holding her down for bloodwork just a few hours back was blown to smithereens while enduring a new version of hell called *ultrasound*. I used my legs to hold hers in place. I held her tiny arms in my hands to keep her from gifting black eyes. I pleaded for answers but the technician kept her gaze on the screen and her lips sewn shut. On the way out of the room she uttered but just a few words, "It'll be okay, I had cancer when I was a kid too."

As if I had just taken a freight train to the stomach, I tried to look back at the technician to beg her for indulgence. But like a ghost in the dead that was this night, she was already gone. Every bit of warmth had left my body, leaving a trail of dying flesh in the hallways meant to preserve life. The only thing that restored my breath was her breath and by the wheels of our new bed, we forged on. We walked down hallways painted with bright colors and childlike dreams, living our nightmare. I stood firm in the entrance of our room for the night. A red, blue and yellow birdcage overpowered the otherwise empty room. I made it very plain that I would not be putting her in the crib, and I got pushback as she stated that there were no other options. I shoved harder this time, noting that I would then be in there with her and not another word was spoken about it. Everyone insisted that I eat or drink, but I was so full already. I was full of fury, fear and desperation, completely broken. All I wanted was to go home, but I had no idea how very far away home was. When my family left, I felt empty and the space around me was suffocating. There were so many people in and out of the room that there was not much space at all. It was like an out-of-body experience. I wasn't even there. I could see myself sitting right next to her as she slept in that cage, a translucent image of who

I was not moments ago. Her nurse was standing at my side and I was begging her to just put me out of my misery. Like a gun kissing my temple, I just wanted someone to pull the damn trigger. I was desperate for an answer and she answered in the best way that she could. I heard her loud and clear. I hadn't swallowed the pill, yet it was on the tip of my tongue, dancing, teasing, bleeding me from the inside out. My eyes never took its gaze away from the night. I was on guard, sword in hand, for whatever demon was up to bat next. With the rise of the sun, the pill had half melted, but I refused to swallow. I was still clinging to that last thread of hope, that maybe this was all just a horrific dream. But as the room filled with more and more people, it was time to wake up.

She had a spinal tap (a needle inserted into her spine extracting spinal fluid) to see if there were cancer cells inside the fluid. She also had a bone marrow biopsy (a needle inserted deep into her bone) to see if there were cancer cells in the marrow. Her doctor entered the room with his head in his chest stating, "There's still a chance this could just be a virus, but I think it is leukemia." Our world shattered like a sledgehammer to a brick wall. We were all in pieces. There is not a glue in existence that could mend this kind of broken. There was a plethora of words followed by that sentence but I couldn't hear a thing. It was like a megaphone had been held to my ear, the word *leukemia* was still blowing out my eardrum. I was nodding my head as if the voice didn't sound like he was speaking in tongues under 80 feet of water. I was still mothering while choking down the reality that she could be dying in my arms. My body had been hosed in nitrogen gas. I was paralyzed. I was trapped inside a plastic bag, my nails shredding to create holes as I was gasping for air. Like a tree holding up its branches, my roots were planted beneath her cage. My trunk sturdy, sure to withstand the next gust of wind on its way. The machines with their endless countdowns and a beeping that makes a fog horn sound like that of a church bell. Her thumb, her only source of self-soothing, was bound by a brace. She would hit herself in the face, attempting to make it all better. I sang the alphabet song, Twinkle Twinkle Little Star and Itsy-bitsy Spider, throwing glitter at the wall in a place that held no shiny. The night birthed hauntings from the depths of the devil's garden. But these weren't ghosts. This was our new reality. I wanted to rip everything off of her, put her in the car and drive away with no GPS, but I couldn't. She was dying in front of me, and the only thing I could do was hold her down, keep her bound, and beg her to breathe.

It's *leukemia*, a word that rips my breath from my lungs. I thought my eardrums had burst yesterday but today this megaphone just took off more than half of my face. With my blood pooling and any piece of life I had left lying on the floor, I said, "I need to get out of here." In the hall, everything looked blurry. I saw fuzzy faces like I was inside one of those strobe light checkered rooms of a haunted house. The walls were closing in on me like an avalanche. I kept repeating, "I need to get out of here." A woman was guiding me through some doors. I don't remember my feet moving or moving my body through the hospital. It felt like my blood sugar had crashed suddenly and I was just moments before passing out. The air hit my face and I gasped so hard I damn near fell over, like a mouth full of salt water tasting the surface. I've never stood so close to death, both physically and metaphorically. I'm still not sure a human is equipped to endure this level of pain. I found the pavement in child's pose, banging my palms against its rough exterior, allowing it to slice me open, praying I'd bleed out right there. My friend brought me to my feet, held me in my nothingness, and led me back to Dakota.

The strongest people I'd ever known were breaking before my eyes. They were avoiding eye contact in every way, holding up the walls but in actuality the walls were holding them up. I handed out apologies like I was handing out tissues. I felt responsible for everyone crumbling around me and I still do. Her oncologist said, "This could very well kill her, but my plan is to cure her. It's going to take every tool in my toolbox but my plan is to cure her." The only physical point worse than where we existed in this moment, would be her death. I said, "I can't live in a world without her." Those words are the truest parts of me. Her death would be my own. My nose crinkled at the smell of my own decay from the inside out. The only chance at her living was to face the very thing attempting to cause her death. I loathed his words, but I clung to them because I trusted him. With his tools in hand, we began to fight for her life.

Leukemia is a blood cancer where the components that make up the blood develop incorrectly, prohibiting the body's ability to fight off infection. Dakota was diagnosed with infantile Pre-B cell Acute Lymphoblastic Leukemia, rare in that it is not a disease that typically affects infants. She would need two years' worth of treatment consisting of harsh 30-year-old chemotherapy drugs and steroids. The kitchen sink is how he referred to it because it is rare that infants respond well to this regimen alone. Most need further, more intense interventions to reach survival. The first goal was to reach MRD negative - minimal residual disease. The steroids alone could take away her cancer, but leukemia is very aggressive. Chemotherapy would hopefully rid it in its entirety. She would need a Broviac, which is tubing lined inside of her to administer her medications on a daily basis, multiple times a day. She would need blood transfusions, platelets, lumbar punctures, and a multitude of other medications to give her a chance at survival. We would need to bring her to the brink of death in order to have a chance at saving her.

Her first blood transfusion gave her an immediate rash. It covered her body in red hives as she let out a shriek like that of a dying rabbit. Or maybe it was the 50 medications that had been pumped into her body after barely having Tylenol for the last six months of her life. The rash faded. The steroids made her inconsolable. I've seen grown men on them that she would put to shame. I had no other choice then, but to hand her over to complete strangers after being informed that she could die. It was nowhere near an easy hand-off and more so a prying from my grip as I begged them to bring her back to me. The Broviac was an image that took me to my knees. I could trace the tubing with my fingertips beneath her fragile, baby-soft skin. White tubes hung out of her like a jellyfish had embedded itself in her chest. After anesthesia, her head fell away from her neck. She cried with such depth her veins threatened to pulse outside of her insides. She was painted black and blue, cherry red from her screams. When I could finally hold her, it took everything in me to continue to stand. Easy would have been assuming the fetal position and pining for a slow death. We had a meeting that lasted from evening into the wee hours of the morning. Her oncologist reinforced that this could take her life, killing us all over again. He reinforced his plan, a roadmap of the climb ahead. All uphill in a little red wagon, a forecast of torrential downpours and 100 mile per hour winds. He handed off a white binder that is still far too heavy for me to pick up. It outlines all of the damage we would be inflicting both in and out of treatment, and short- and long-term effects. Her cancer was not the only threat. The treatment is so grueling, it alone could take her life. She would lose her hair and her ability to take anything by mouth, including food and drink. She would feel sick more often than not and infections, even as slight as the common cold, could cause her death. The drugs could stunt her growth, cause infertility, heart defects, neurological and psychological deficits. She could endure memory loss, seizures, physical ailments. The lists are endless. But this was necessary to give her a chance at life, to keep her alive. I couldn't wrap my head around the letters on the pages, like staring into alphabet soup. They were just words at the time, distorted black images on paper that was far too white. I kept thinking this man was supposed to be home with his wife, yet here he was, answering every question as if we were sharing stories and having drinks. He said he would try to save my daughter, to cure her, and I believed him. I walked outside with a family member as he begged me to hold on to hope. As I was walking away from him, I felt I had let him down. I was failing everyone around me. My fingertips were barely touching the tip of the cliff and I couldn't catch my grip. My body was flailing above the rocks, their sharp edges taunting me, calling me to succumb to my death. I let go and fell through the sky. The thin air was kissing my burnt flesh the entire way down. The crash into the earth was glorious. It relieved the incurable pain that could only be healed by death. I died that day, clinging to her breath, for the will to survive.

She received dexamethasone in the morning and again at night, every single day. It made her skin lobster red, as if she had been lathered in baby oil basking in the sun. She was puffed up like the marshmallow man who could barely navigate the kitchen in the commercial. She would let out screams that made my own throat ache. I could hear the raw in her tonsils. No matter how close I held her, she was undeniably miserable to put it kindly. She only wanted to be held, and the holder had to be in standing. She would fall asleep for brief durations, 20 to 30 minutes at a time. If there was an attempt to sit, she would wake in protest and scream for hours. Steroids are known to cause joint pain, heat spells, a bottomless hunger and stomach pain. As an infant, she couldn't tell us what she was feeling. Her only form of making us aware of her pain and discomfort was to cry out in hopes that we'd help her find some relief. But there was nothing we could do. Tylenol would mask fevers and chemotherapy made her immunocompromised. A fever would be an indication of an infection. Therefore, we were limited in what we could give her for pain. I was failing her with every swing and a miss. The punching bag was hitting my face harder than any punch I had laid into it.

I was covered in bruises, both visible and invisible. I was at war with my thoughts, my heart and my body was shedding skin by the minute. I was standing entangled by a web of tubing filled

15

with poison, with my baby in my arms. Hell's creatures were grabbing for her at my feet while I bounced her and sang nursery rhymes. My soul was in the corner of the room, curled into herself screaming at the top of her lungs, with a muzzle over her mouth. She was blanketed in her own fire and her breath alone made the flames kiss the ceiling. Dakota would lift her head from my left shoulder to find my gaze. She would search my eyes for comfort and assurance. I had absolutely nothing to give her, but I gave her every ounce of me. She would find brief periods of rest where I could lay her down in the cage and sprint for the bathroom. There, I would muster the courage to meet my gaze in the reflection in the mirror. It was an appalling site as I had no idea who was looking back at me. Her eyes were empty, her nose was curved to the left and her smile was nonexistent. I couldn't help but bathe my face in my wet grief, ashamed and attempting to find grace in the same space. With my shoulders wrapped 20 times over my eyebrows, I looked at the dead girl looking back me and I asked her, "What would you say to Dakota?"

I told her, I would say, "I fight for you baby girl, every second of every day. Even when I have nothing left, I am fighting for you. Words are powerful and they can make us or break us. We have heard enough words in the last two weeks to destroy an army with a whisper. We have no other choice but to stand together, strong, worn, tired but fighting. Sometimes you need to speak love into yourself. Your own words can be the last drop of strength you need to get up. We are the muscle we need to find our footing and wipe away our tears so we can open the door and smile back at the world. So we can face the darkness with sunshine and a power like no other. We have to beat all the bad words with good ones. Encouragement is power, not just for others, but for ourselves too. The more positive words we speak, the better chance we have at changing the world. Dakota, you were born to change the world. Your spirit is far stronger than anyone I know. You fight with a smile that is an unstoppable force. I am right here, fighting with you. I will never leave you. Together, we got this." With oceans layering my face, I made a choice I never could have imagined would have been a choice. When a girl can't change her situation, she changes her appearance. I decided to physically showcase the invisible loss I was enduring. Strand by strand, I chose to shave my head.

With Dakota in my lap and my mom behind me, I could hear the buzzer purring. It was surreal to feel the clippers against my scalp. It was physically metaphoric watching my blonde locks fall to the floor. Dakota was watching in awe and confusion. My mom was more emotional as she made note she hadn't seen my head in a very long time. I could feel the weight decreasing with each clump that waterfalled in front of my face. It was beyond therapeutic in that it was giving a chosen change to my changes that had no choices. It was symbolic in giving physical representation to the emotional loss I had been enduring in these last few days. It was for me, facing my demons, my fears, my pain and one of my many deaths. It gave voice to the words my tongue couldn't speak. It was acceptance of my rebirth, washing myself in her blood. I couldn't endure this for her, but I would suffer in every way I possibly could with her. I rubbed my new fuzzy head with my hand and laughed as it reminded me of my fascination I had with my brother's shaved head as a child. I took Dakota's hands and put them on my head. She looked shocked and in wonder. I cried in this moment because my new fuzzy head was explaining to her that I was with her to the nth degree. With her on my hip, I found my reflection once again. I didn't know this girl either, but I adored her badassery. Our bruises became our war paint and we were dressed to fight.

My eyes were swollen shut from the blind hits and lack of sleep. In a matter of days, I was told my daughter had cancer that could cause her death. We gave up our home as we were informed that we would be living inside the hospital more than we would not. I was attempting to decide what to do about my career and I was now not just a mother, but a caregiver. I was struggling like an elephant sinking to the ocean floor, barricaded inside a net wrapped in barbed wire with tiger sharks circling. I pitied anyone who may have crossed my flame-filled path. I made my plea just after I had wiped my baby down with disinfectant wipes, the form of a bath given in a hospital to prevent germs from taking your child's life before cancer does. I simply stated that when the body is run down, rest is best. But she couldn't find rest as she was constantly being poked and prodded. Therefore, her healing and recovery was constantly being put on pause. I could see sympathy in their eyes as their mouths spoke of job requirements. In a professional manner, I understood, but as a mother I was spitting fireballs. I have no doubt they had "bless your heart" names for me and played "not it" games when the light above our door would flash. I don't blame them at all.

At home, we would lay wrapped up in one another on the

couch. At the hospital, it was mandatory that she sleep in the crib. I would take the couch and daddy would take the floor. She was feeling beyond awful. She could barely keep her head up. She held a soft cry even in her sleep, and her body was writhing as if it were being eaten alive by thousands of spiders. I pulled her into me on the couch and like a mama bear nestled deep inside a cave, we found rest within one another. A nurse came in and tapped me on my arm. She said, "Mom, you have to put the baby in the crib." Every ounce of sanity I had left flew out of the window like blown dust. The chains broke, windows shattered, the wind gusts poured in and the room was engulfed in flames within seconds.

I said, "She has cancer. She doesn't feel good and I'm not leaving her." She said she understood but it was policy. I told her I didn't care. She told me she could lose her job. I told her I could lose my daughter. She left the room and I felt like scum. My skin was oozing with baby cobras and vile green vomit. I couldn't stand my own disgusting stench. I immediately wanted to apologize and retract every drop of venom I had spewed. My words were horrific, but they held a disgusting truth. With my tail between my legs, I apologized the following morning. There's no way to know how you'll react until you're in the moment begging for a reaction. We were drifting in the storm, surfing on a wooden door. The shoreline was barely a speck in our line of vision. We couldn't remember anything we were told as our ears were still ringing from the word *leukemia*. We were just trying not to drown, making every attempt to save her in the midst of our treading water. We didn't see the tsunami headed straight for us. It barely made a sound. The days ahead slowly chipped away at the remainder our souls. The chains broke, windows shattered, and the wind gusts poured in. The room resembled hell within seconds.

The chipping away was caused by a word that haunts me daily. Mucositis is a cluster of blisters that form and spread throughout the digestive tract, a side effect from chemotherapy. They resemble cauliflower heads and feel like burns in the mouth. They started inside Dakota, beyond what we could see. She began to refuse food and drink as drool would pour from the side of her lips. Her diaper area looked as if a torch was held to it. We began using a regimen called concrete, which is layering her private areas in a paste to decrease the amount of chemicals coming in contact with her skin to prevent further chemical burns. Her cheeks were that of a chipmunk stuffed with steroids. Her belly round and hard, giving Buddha a run for his money. Her weight was dropping from lack of food intake. Her team began discussing a feeding tube with me because if her nutrition was not upheld, she would become weak and it would become more difficult for her to fight. I fought it like hell because I'm the mom who wants her to do as much as she can on her own. May it be a disgusting form of tough love or a complete mom fail, both would be more than accurate. I was barely treading water in uncharted waters and I had absolutely no clue what I was doing. Her team discussed pain management medications to help provide her some comfort. I'm not a medicine person by any means. Up until this point I could count on one hand how many times I had given Dakota Tylenol. They told me quite a few times that she was in pain. I felt she had already had so much medicine running through her body that I didn't want to add insult to injury.

She was wailing, a cry that made my shoulders blanket my ears and my blood run cold for over six hours. Her bottom was covered in open blisters and her mouth looked like it was caked in cottage cheese. Human design continued on despite the body battling cancer as she was cutting teeth too. I caved and asked that she receive something to ease her pain, but it was too late. Her pain was beyond a ten out of ten. I had let my baby suffer tremendously. The Benadryl made her have seizure-like activity, an adverse reaction. Her eyes would lock and her body would flail like a baby bird attempting to fly. She would shake as if she were naked out in sub degree temperatures. The Tylenol didn't touch her, so our next option was morphine. My infant was on morphine. If I hadn't longed for the sweet bliss of plummeting to my death before, I more than longed to taste it now. She was placed on TPN (total parenteral nutrition), an IV that provides her body with nutrition. We hadn't hit bottom just yet. It would only get worse before it would get better. This was just one of the many moments I couldn't fathom any worse, but worse was already on its way. Then her central line stopped giving blood return. I'd hold her in different positions in attempts to help the blood flow. She was seated in my lap with her arms up, then down. I'd place her on her side moving her arms in circles. I had to force her on her back with her arms up, being sure she didn't choke on the blood pouring from her mouth. There was still no blood coming from her line. Without her blood, we didn't have counts. Without her numbers, we didn't know where her body stood in her battle. Without knowing if she was standing in her fight or on her knees, she

21

could die. Kicking her while she was down, the war couldn't stop. She began receiving some of the most powerful forms of chemotherapy. She was grinding her teeth due to the pain and her loose stools were making it almost impossible to keep from peeling back layers of skin. We figured out how to get her inside an infant jumping chair, making failed attempts at normalcy. Even games were short lived as she was feeling something awful and barely pushing through her pain. Her team was growing in numbers with wound care, an optometrist and an entire pediatric physician team stepping up to the plate. All hands were on deck. Sleep was almost non-existent for all three of us as our door was ever revolving. She was already on all fours attempting to stand with blood pouring from her mouth, but cancer was still raging inside of her. We had to continue to take our shots at the enemy, knowing damn well it would push her body to that fine line. If we didn't press on, she could die. If we continued to throw punches, she could die. Without numbers, she could die. Our options were limited in keeping her alive. Our spirits were scraping the depths of the earth. Our days were relentless in testing every ounce of effort we had to give. Our nights were spent inside the barrel of the under tow, like spinning in a washing machine. We would hold our breath awaiting the rise of the sun, to catapult ourselves to the surface in search of air. Crawling out of our skin, as there was no escape from our living hell. She reached monthly milestones encased inside four walls with only a window to see outside of our world. Every minute was celebrated as just a few weeks ago we were told we were racing the clock.

The clock ticked on. Mother's Day came and went, but not

without a slap in the face. My husband, being the man he is, brought flowers to our hospital room. I remember my heart fluttered and sank all in the same moment, as flowers were now a danger to Dakota. He could see the anguish in my face and my words crushed his soul. A feather could have flattened him, and I was his ten-ton hammer. Everything that had been so normal, even something as simple as the kind gesture of a flower, was now life-threatening. She wasn't awake much and when she was, she was projectile vomiting. Her blood pressure began running too high and she had started a runny nose. She was on fluids as she wasn't eating and drinking, but her tiny body had ballooned and her skin became so stretched it was shiny. I would take a walk every once in a while, something so simple that became a luxury. Living on the inside, I would forget the warm kiss of the sun and the hug of a summer breeze. My stroll was only 20 minutes or so at a time. But the space outside of our space gave me a breath to go back in and the bravery to continue to breathe. Dakota's line had to be fixed, which meant surgery. Her Broviac had stopped giving blood return, which meant there was a problem on the inside. In the battle against leukemia, numbers are our lifeline. They tell the story of the things we cannot see - if we are close to a win or facing down a potential punch to the gut. At this point she had pupil dilation and a droopy eye, and blood pressure was all over the place. An ultrasound of the kidneys had to be performed as her output wasn't great and she was retaining so much fluid. An MRI needed to be done to see if there were any other underlying issues that we were missing. The arrows were pointing in all directions with no definite answer. Surgery was our only option. Once she was deemed well enough, they would remove her original Broviac from the

23

left side of her chest and place a new one on the right side. We were on a stretcher headed down to ultrasound. I was telling her it was okay while lying through my teeth as none of this is okay. We were on a rollercoaster through endless hallways with temperatures that make a meat freezer feel like a popsicle day in August. I loathe ultrasounds. I held her down with my legs and restrained her arms with my own. Sweat mixed with our tears, and we were both a salty wet mess. Time moves excruciatingly slow, with every second ticking by like a year. Her eyes searched for mine, begging me to make it stop. My heart bled out on the floor with guilt. There were tons of other people around, which was poison for Dakota. I blanketed her in my sweater in my failed attempts to protect her, in every way, every day, I felt as if I were failing her.

They put her under anesthesia for the MRI. Seeing her after anesthesia was like looking at your child after their first fight in fight club. Her body was battered, a mind trick as if she were lifeless. She was gray in color and painted with deep purple bruises. Her eyes were closed, but she still let out her screams. Her body was immoveable, but she could not stop squirming. She longed for my arms, but we weren't permitted to hold one another. I would pet her skin through the steel bars and barbed wire. It was imprisonment for both of us in every way. After 30 minutes, we were granted an embrace. I had to hold her head in place because it was as if a puppet master were on the floor getting his kicks from yanking the back of her skull from her neck. She would crawl up my body like a cub scales a tree. Her body would give off heat like a desert. She made every attempt to flee the demons who were coming for her, but they had already infiltrated. She was exhausted, yet she couldn't sleep. Tylenol would help, but she would continue to let out a soft whimper in her rest. It was absolute torture to watch my baby sit atop a rooftop that was engulfed in flames. It defeated me as I was bound in a cage 50 feet away. A hooded man would tap a baseball bat against the metal that surrounded me. He'd whisper sweet nothings directly from the serpent's tongue as he sprayed gasoline through the firehose. Death would have been a lavender bubble bath with rose petals, and I awaited its ambiance with open arms.

Like a 70-pound warrior layered in 100 pounds of armor, still swinging an ironclad sword, we rose the following day. On the docket, was a routine spinal tap and surgery for a new Broviac placement. During her surgery, I visited the clinic as this would be our second home to our fifth-floor stay. It was like a scene like no horror film could ever depict. It looked fun and playful, enticing in some dark alley lollipop kind of way. It was smeared with bright colors and a big tree right in the center. Children were reclined with poison being pumped into their veins. Arts and crafts were on the table next to blue vomit bags. It was the loveliest most vile place I had ever seen. I held it together while I was in there, but I damn near fell to the floor out in the hallway, gasping for breath. My heart broke for every child that was forced to live this life. Selfishly, it was one of the first times I had admitted to myself that this was in fact, our life.

We waited in the basement-like room filled with tapping feet and an anxiousness that made banging your head on the wall seem sane. Even Gandhi couldn't find Zen there. The waiting was like being inside a block of ice on city streets at Spring, melting one drop at a time but not nearly fast enough. Finally, we were called back where the surgeon drew a diagram to show his work inside our baby. Her line was moved to the other part of her chest. More holes in my infant. He said to wait just 15 to 20 more minutes. An hour had gone by and I knew in my gut something was wrong. We were called back again and he told us something had happened. She couldn't breathe on her own after the anesthesia. When they removed the tube from her throat, she had turned purple from her chest up and they had to intubate again so she could breathe. My baby was now vented in the PICU. If a cat has nine lives, I was a damn lion because I had just died again.

CHAPTER 2

$\mathcal{W}$e were escorted down meat freezer like hallways that held the secret sobs of many a mother's heart. We walked through giant metal doors that lead to our unknown, longing to sprint to her. Our feet barely moved as we were paralyzed by fear of the condition she may be in. We entered yet another room to sit and wait. I physically couldn't sit. I just paced back and forth. I saw our social worker in the hall and I ran to her, fell into her. She heard me without my voice breaking a whisper. She felt the heaviness of my heart, listened to the gasping of my breath and held me as I crumbled to the floor. She knew exactly where I stood in this place as she herself wears shoes like mine. I returned to the room as a team of doctors flooded in. They asked me to sit down, but I still couldn't sit. They spoke words that sounded like muffles of conversation at an outside concert despite standing side-by-side. They had no answers as to how we ended up here and they smiled politely through their delivery of worst-case scenarios. I was barely treading water, nodding my head, attempting to mask my drowning while the walls caved in. After words like pulmonary embolism, which was ruled out, they finally whispered the words I was longing to hear: "You can go back to see her."

The PICU is different, like black coffee ground from dirt in the shoe of a corpse. Chaotic, like a 50-car pile-up on the highway at rush hour after school lets out. The noise is deafening. Focus is a lost cause on the brain attempting to process the black Friday mayhem and the ringing from the shotguns firing. I squinted my eyes as if wrinkling my forehead would somehow calm this side of crazy. It's all business and no emotion. Not a smile or a tear. Just dead eyes and empty souls.

Children are facing down death 30 rooms deep. There is not a millimeter of space for human emotion. I finally reached her room, but turning the corner from the hallway to her doorway was like coming face to face with the devil's breath. Nothing in this world prepares you for a sight like that, to see your child knocking on death's door. There were people all around her bed making it difficult for my eyes to find her. She looked lifeless, big tubes protruding from her face. Tape was glued to her cheeks. Huge purple bruises blanketed her neck and chest. Her skin had no color and she was so swollen, her veins were a roadmap showcasing her fight. I wasn't allowed to touch her, so I put myself in the corner. I broke like a looming storm cloud releasing its wrath on the earth below. It felt like I was being ripped to shreds like a tree deep inside of a chipper. Every piece of me wanted to run to her and hold her close. I wanted to apologize and promise to never leave her again. I was silently thanking her for coming back. My gaze never lost sight of her and with the thought of her finding breath again, I slowly found my own. The nurse turned to me and said, "Mom are you okay?" I was taken aback by the question as I couldn't comprehend how that could even be a question. I had no words, yet my tongue mustered up the strength to whisper, "No, I am not okay."

I wasn't alone in the broken for long as family began trickling in one by one. Each person broke at the sight of what shouldn't be seen. It was like we were lining up execution style, taking bullet after bullet, falling to the ground but fighting to stay standing. We would talk to her, tell her we love her and that we were here. When I rubbed her head, her hair started falling out all over the pillow. My chest tightened as if I had just taken a direct hit from an 18-wheeler to my sternum. My hands shook at the physical visual of what was now our reality. I was in the fetal position screaming at the top of my lungs inside, but with people all around me, I bit down hard and refused to let a tear fall. In the same way they entered, they left one by one. My husband had to find another room in the hospital to sleep in as only one parent was allowed in the room overnight. We were divided in every way possible, yet we needed one another more than ever. It was just Dakota and me, alone in a space that gives *lonely* an entirely new definition. She was embedded in sheets that matched her skin tone, immobilized in every sense of the word. Her body read me the story of what happened while we were apart while her eyes asked me questions I had no answers for. I sat beside her crib apologizing relentlessly, singing a melody to the drum of the beeping, like heavy metal in a soundproof room. The night, like an underground tunnel, knows no light or end.

The arrival of the morning light brought a flood of people in the room, forcing my burning eyes to widen and find full gaze. The swarm of white jackets decided that they were going to take the tube out to see if she could breathe on her own. They warned us of the multitude of outcomes, including her airway closing and the possibility of immediate re-intubation. We nodded our heads in agreement that the potential reward outweighed the risk and we aligned ourselves at the foot of her bed. We were cheering her on as if we were at a football game and the quarterback was gunning for a touchdown. Bodies surrounded hers, and like hands on a hose, they were pulling the tube slathered in her secretions out from inside her. Her mouth opened and she let out this faint, aching, raspy, hail Mary cry. It was like the moment she was born again, her first breath for the second time.

I asked immediately to hold her, but I was still not allowed despite her needing our embrace the most. We stood there listening to her cry this ache that stole the beat of our hearts. We were all holding our breath for her as they began a series of tests to ensure that her breathing was no longer in danger. Finally, I was granted permission to do what feels most natural to me. I climbed on a step stool because I am the size of a 12-year-old. I found my way to her through the web of tubing and wires and for the first time since she almost left me, I held my baby. I ugly cried while shaking like a leaf. I felt hands on me to be sure we didn't fall, but I was so focused on stitching us back together, deleting any seams. We were on limited time. Just as she began to settle in my arms, I had to put her back down. I had to tear us apart again because, rules. It was like ripping off a limb, more so like detaching the soul from the human body. She wailed and although I was beyond grateful for her voice, I was consumed with fury being apart from her again. The distance acting as gasoline, I was twitching like a lone piece of paper in a tornado. She was screaming uncontrollably and I held my tongue for a few short minutes. Then I asked, more so stated, "If you let me hold her, maybe she'll calm down." Even rules bend sometimes and like butter we melted into one other. She wasn't put back in that bed until the evening fell. We were separated again but closer than ever, holding onto the scent of one another. Daddy was finding sleep in his car as we were wishing away the ocean of demons between us. Our tears spoke the words our lips couldn't whisper. She was breathing, giving us breath through her breath. It was yet another sleepless night in which we both fought to stay above the darkness. The morning brought light. We were leaving the PICU.

Leaving meant revealing the damage that had been done. They removed the tubing and the tape. I could see the effects of losing breath on her skin. I could visibly see the touch of poison seeping through her pores and I had never felt like more of a failure in my life. My tongue couldn't find the words to express my apologies. I was desperate for her to know how deeply sorry I was. Drowning in my grief, I climbed into her crib. I knew I wasn't allowed, but I didn't care. I needed her to know that I was there and that I'd never fail her again. The nurses reiterated the rules and I eventually complied, but not without every attempt to convince them otherwise. Arriving back on the fifth floor was like going home or the closest recollection I had of what that was like. Once we were settled in to yet another room, I crawled back into my true home, right beside her. The nurses let me stay because up there, human emotion is tolerated. Before the evening fell, I asked one of her nurses to grab me a pair of scissors. She sat there with me in a moment no mother should ever know. I cut Dakota's hair as I did not want her to experience that loss piece by piece. My pain-filled eyes made it difficult to see, but with her angel beside me, I mothered in a way I didn't know I was capable of. I was breaking all of the rules but remaining exactly where I was meant to be. Hope was on the horizon if I could convince her to take in a few ounces of milk by mouth. I started with a syringe which she fought at first, but eventually with an enormous amount of cheerleading, she was taking in an ounce here and there before the evening came.

With the arrival of the morning, she had some ounces down with new hair to boot and we were leaving. But not without one last kick in the pants from chemo as the war continued to rage on. For the first time in well over a month, we would walk through the doors that put a period on our before. Catching the wings of a jet wouldn't be fast enough. I learned to be her nurse outside of the hospital. I was no longer just a mom, but now a caregiver. I was sure to cross our T's and dot our I's, but then panic set in. My face was buried in a paper bag searching for air at the thought of the remanence of life outside of this life. The world was nothing short of a deathtrap now and Dakota and I hadn't been out there since the before. If I placed her back in my womb it wouldn't suffice. An army of Navy SEALs wouldn't have the strength to handle this job. I couldn't drive as I was physically and mentally incapable of focusing on anything outside of keeping her alive. She cried the whole way and I did too. The two of us were so unsure of which world was more devouring, out there or in there. I couldn't understand how people were driving around us as if my child weren't fighting for her life in the backseat of the car. We made it, "home", my parents' home. Our home, along with the life we had known, was long gone. It was immediate shock seeing our life in boxes stacked in the garage. Our before stacked high in front of me was the visual of the pause button. I was so overwhelmed, my skin was itching with invisible hives. A hot shower helped, but I could still feel the lumps. It would have been better if the skin had melted from the bone. Sitting on that shower floor didn't come close to the depths of the hell I was swimming in. It felt like I was living in a nightmare and in fact, I was. I didn't know how to settle in. There was no place to settle. Every bit of our life was in limbo, like balls floating in the abyss, taunting each other to drop. We stood in the wait with boxes, duffle bags and go bags, forcing ourselves to not move an inch, out of fear of what the next hour could bring. Home-cooked meals were nice when I had the energy to bring food to my mouth. I felt guilty for going outside as I made attempts to befriend the sun. Her shine was outcasted by the clouds hovering inches above my head, reminding me that Dakota couldn't be with me. Even life's smallest pleasures encased me in darkness. Insomnia was an enemy who never left as we were all accustomed to the constant interruption. The three of us in the same bed, fighting off the terrors of the night. Four days came and went in a blink. It was time to pack up and leave again. Going back made it real, solidified this death of life. As the doors closed behind us this time, we were in the know that we may not come back out.

We arrived back at the hospital, our new home away from home. She was weighed, height-checked, and her ankle bracelets were already placing her on hospital arrest before I could even blink. Our clothes were unpacked as if we had done this before but she didn't make counts. This cancer life is a numbers game and I'll be the first to tell you I suck at numbers. The doctor said words at a sprinter's speed, but my brain was overwhelmed with horrific thoughts and moved at a snail's pace. Chemotherapy had wiped out her bone marrow which was a job well done. In our strategy to battle cancer, we wanted this to happen. This was where we were to wait for her body to recover in order to continue knocking her down, in hopes that at some point, we would beat her cancer. If that doesn't make sense, pull up a chair, because it still doesn't make sense to me. No chemo means pay over two hundred dollars, pass go and go home. I didn't even know what the hell home meant anymore. Just as we began to repack what had been unpacked, her oncologist noticed her right cheek was swollen and so tight it was shiny. Everything sounds the alarms. Because she was immunocompromised and at a high risk for infection, we were granted a one-way ticket to admission. No treatment meant cancer can grow. Cancer growing means she could die. She could have been dying, right before our eyes, again. Once again, we were a long way from home.

We left our clothes in the drawers and deflated in our defeat on the couch. There was no irony that it began raining outside, giving a visual in correspondence with the storms we were enduring inside. Viral panels were run and more antibiotics flowed through just in case something was in fact brewing in her already worn little body. Thankfully it was an uneventful short stay and within two days, we were able to once again, pack up and head home. It was nice to not be there, to lay in the same bed without getting in trouble. To move around without being bound by a pole and having more than four walls to venture, but I was haunted. The time at home was a window left wide open during a tornado warning and we were just sitting ducks in the attic. But going back meant purposely making her violently ill and bringing her body far too close to death in hopes of keeping her from actually dying. This is the very essence of the unspoken definition to screw with the human mind. The following day, we were up to bat for numbers. With no helmet on our heads or cleats on feet, no matter if we struck out or hit a homerun, we were guaranteed to get hit with the ball. If counts were made, we would begin pumping her with poison. If her body wasn't ready, we would be heading home to welcome cancer with balloons and confetti to take her life. I was on a rollercoaster ride vomiting all day long because this time, I knew what was coming. I could smell the toxins that were to course through her veins. I was holding onto her smile selfishly for my own will to live as I knew it was about to fade. I barely let her feet touch the floor as I was having a premonition of the collision up ahead. I heard the cracking of her bones. Her screams were the ghost's boo I couldn't escape. I was desperately trying to be a heavy-duty air bag on all sides, but I was barely measuring up to a cheap plastic grocery bag at most. I was standing on the side of the road, listening to the screech of the brakes. It was coming and there was not a damn thing I could do about it. It wasn't a choice. It was the necessary evil. The only way to have any chance at giving her life was to damn near kill her. With her head molded into my chest, I was whispering into the night, "You can't have her you bastard!" His gas-like breath on my neck, begging me to gamble, I rolled the dice praying for sixes.

I lost count at how many times I had yelled at the sky in those first few weeks. There were countless times I had fallen to the ground beneath me, crawled into dark places inside myself that I didn't know existed, begging Him to make this all go away. Despite the depths of my agony, I still believed. I do not believe He is a cruel God, but a God who loves His children, a Creator who would never do anything to hurt all that He loves. I have faith that He loves us always and carries us when we are too weak to take another step. I believe His plan is far greater than ours at any given time despite the inability as humans to see as He sees. In no way does any of this mean that I have not been angry, confused, hurt beyond measure, broken without repair and utterly defeated. At times it felt as if He had let the devil win at our expense. My daughter may or may not live. Her childhood here on earth has been nothing short of captivity and a brutal uphill battle no child should know. I am angry every day but He is still good. I know in my heart He will see us through as He has countless times. Through Dakota's journey He has brought non-believers to their knees. It is His most exquisite work in its purest form. When she smiled through the pain, laughed through the hurt and hugged so hard as if she were attempting to love it all away, that was Him. I continued to yell to Him on a daily basis. I screamed out unto to the sky, "Where are you?" Instead of striking my human self down, He embraced me in His love, giving me strength in my weakness. My faith was tested daily, but His love was our steady. We were forever adrift on a piece of carboard in the storm, but holding on as He continued to hold us.

We walked into a giant room with colorful walls and a big tree in the middle. There were kind faces with warm smiles and hot cocoa-esque greetings. All the fluff in attempts to mask the pale children walking around with their pole in tow and poison coursing through their blood. It was a sight not even hell's serpent tongue could explain. It was heartbreaking to see children so broken, frail, deflated, yet fighting for their lives. Although they were not mine, I wanted to cradle them and take their boo boos away, protect them, even though I couldn't. I now knew that just my touch could kill them. I realized the ambulance lights I myself couldn't break my stare of, were the same lights projecting from behind the curtain hanging in front of us. This place was the road and we were the scene of the accident. There were moments when her laugh distracted me from everyone's eyes. But as the chaos continued to spin in cycle, it hit me like a steel barrel to my gut - this was our world now. It took everything in me not to crawl out of my skin and beeline it to the exit. I sat with Dakota in my lap, reading stories, smiling through the grind of my teeth. We were on borrowed time, yet the second hand felt like an eternity. I made attempts to think outside of the here and now, fantasizing about her first birthday, her fifth birthday. But with bile drying out the roof of my mouth, at the too honest truth, that we may not make it to those parties. I assume the loss of color in my face and the salt water droplets around my feet caught some attention, as we were told they would change her dressing and we were to exit and wait.

We found ourselves in yet another room where women were masked and gloved. Silver tables adorned with needles, tubes and bandages. Dakota was already a brutal shade of red. I was assisting in the hog tying. I loathed this octave of her shrill. I covered her mouth with a mask and my hand as my other hand held back her swings. My legs kept her legs from kicking and everyone was sweating. They attempted to distract her with *Paw Patrol* and songs but she refused any of our shenanigans. They had to peel back the tape and the dressing from her fragile skin. The tape burned her skin like a cigarette to flesh. Once the dressing was removed, the area was lathered in cleaning products to decrease risk of infection, as there was always an open hole inside her chest just begging for death to seep in. She thrashed her body back like an exorcism in rebut. They waved their hands over her wet skin in attempts to speed up the mayhem. Everything used to keep her safe was wet and cold. Snakes would feel like a warm blanket compared to a dressing change. She was barely seven months old at this point and none of this made sense to me, let alone to her. This must have been the sweetest side of hell in her mind. Once everything was dry, they applied a dry dressing to her skin, applying more tape to be sure there were no open spaces for specks of dirt to crawl in and threaten her life. She fell into my shoulder, inserted her thumb and all was right in her world again.

Our feet moved through the red exit and outside to wait for our car. There is a garden outside of the children's cancer center, a physical oxymoron, life within the death. We were alone so I permitted us both to indulge in the gift of the little things. The dangers of grass, dirt and the sun birthed more wrinkles in my forehead. All we now knew was confinement and isolation. We were bubble girls. My eyes welled because I began falling in love with the way the sun was kissing her skin. But my fear grew stronger than my desire to know the taste of love. Oh, but the gentle caress of the breeze with her. I was always treading space between exposing her to life's life and shielding her from death. The yellow of the daffodils begged to be touched. It broke my heart to think her little hands may never hold one. Thank God the car pulled up to save me from my insanity. We drove to the in-between to find more waiting and pacing. The phone rang with failure, still no dice. I leaned up against the wall, caked in defeat. My sails caved in and my balloon collapsed. "Stay home," the voice said, but I couldn't find home if I tried. Here, not there, meant cancer could grow. Cancer growing meant she could leave here. I succumbed to my tears and crashed into the floor with her. We curled into one another, the snuggle that holds the power to heal all of the boo boos. I was attempting to find my way back to the only place that gives me any sense of feeling alive - safe in her arms. More waiting for treatment to take her piece by piece, like a mirror with no luck. For cancer to rear its ugly grin, threatening the few inches left of her life. Desperately begging myself to muster the strength, to peel ourselves off of the floor. To find Bambi legs in standing and continue swinging.

I was standing and swinging while on my knees with my hands behind my back. *Normal* is a word we will never know again. Our lives changed in an instant. We changed on a dime. We will never be who we were and there is no going back. When people would ask how we were, there was a forever pause and a half ass smirk. Just as people do not know what to say to us, we do not know what to say to others. There are no words. Our baby was battling cancer. I am certain those words should not create a sentence. There is not a damn thing normal about those words and there are no words to explain the hell we were enduring on the inside. Everything was a broken puzzle with the pieces themselves broken and scattered all over the floor, and for shits and giggles a giant wind gust had just blown through. Even on our "good days," it was all a mess. We understand that it is impossible to understand. We were in it and we still don't understand. Unless you wear shoes like ours, there is no way to remotely understand. I still pray daily that no one knows what we know, or sees the sites of hell that we have seen. There is no way to endure this death in life and come out alive. There is not a drop of sanity that exists in this insanity. The only way through this is to lose everyone and everything in hopes to not lose your child. This includes yourself. We didn't choose any of this, but we had to become who we needed to be to give her a chance at survival. None of this is anywhere near normal but it is and will forever be our normal.

Our "normal" at "home" consisted of making 10 different varieties of smoothies and 20 different meals before nine a.m. in attempts to encourage her to eat. She had started to develop an aversion to food, anything coming to her mouth, in fear of it causing pain. We spent a lot of time singing songs, reading books, and she fell in love with the movie *Moana*. All of the little things became larger than life because we didn't know how much life we had left. Every moment was precious. Sleep was a chore as insomnia was something we were all suffering through.

It helped to have a piece of our before, our German Shepherd, Chief. He had always been so attentive and protective of her. To her, he was a giant bear. We would enjoy the luxury of a bath together, the space to move about and quite different from cold wet cloths. To find rest together in one space was a utopian dream despite the no sleep, as the three of us needed one another now more than ever and we were apart more often than not. Home was a place for us to pick up pieces of pieces knowing all too well we'd never be whole. It was our in-between, between two dwellings. At times it was far too quiet and it made the noise inside us all the more loud. Other times, it was like a cage inside of a cage, for there was too much space yet never enough. It was a constant reminder of our pause and like chocolate dangling just outside of the window, but melting before we could ever find a taste. It was everything we needed too far out of reach filled with a binding love that *knows no bounds,* but we had become accustomed to war. That is the very essence of the fairness in love and war. The war must be fought with love to stand a chance at a win, but love must be lost to overcome the war.

The casualties of war are often surprising and blindsiding. I was organizing her clothes when I got hit from behind, one hell of a blow. I began to tackle the mountains of our life piled high in the garage. But I was a rookie running in heels with tissues for padding and taking me down would require nothing more than a gentle memory. I was sorting through her clothes from the before, the ones I had intentions for and the new ones that had been donated. I was holding the very clothes I held her in without having any inclination that she had cancer. It was a blade slicing through my insides and I was holding the handle. I was letting go of the swim suits and all too constricting summer clothes I had set my dreams on for our adventures on sunny days. Like a soft blow of lips to a wish on stem, my romantic walks on the beach were washed away with the tide. I was grieving the fantasy of these pretty-in-pink ensembles that served no purpose in our world but had every intention of bringing sparkle to cloudy days. I had a flashback of an afternoon when I was walking towards the cafeteria while we were inpatient. There was a beautiful little girl with golden blonde hair, twirling in a light blue dress. With a sad smile painted on my face, I wondered if my girl would ever get the chance to look like that. On autopilot, I continued to build a pile that could hold her lines yet allow accessibility. I embodied a robot with no capability of emotion until the foam spilled over the top and my boiling water antagonized the flames. At the sight of her dedication gown, I was gasoline being poured over a well-lit forest fire. I broke like porcelain family heirlooms' kiss to a concrete wall. I couldn't choke down another drop of agony. The dam released behind my eyes. My chest succumbed to every memory of our dead before. Embarrassed by my weakness and disgusted by my vulnerability, I covered my face with my child-like hands as if it could hide my raging storm. My head fell back in protest, longing to scream at the ceiling, begging the paint to crack. I threw in the towel, giving the universe the win. I found my way back to the only promise I could still physically hold onto - her in the now. Pulling her in close, I was hopeful for the night and praying for another shot at tomorrow. The war was relentless and even with an end date in sight, there was no end in sight. Life was dead all around me as I stood upon the mountain of what once held so much breath. Huddled together in the center of the ash, love was still forging on.

I took a walk that entailed the greatest distance she and I had had in well over a month. No sooner than my feet started down the driveway, was I consumed with a suffocating guilt. I should not be gifted the nibble of the sweet indulgences she cannot yet taste. Yet the sun beckoned me, making me feel shiny in my dull, like glitter in a swamp. I stretched my arms out, extending the welcome of a hug to the breeze. She began flirting with me with her butterfly kisses. The day smelled of honeysuckles and childhood. I embraced the quiet my soul longed for and my heart found a pace it had forgotten. Chief was at my side, the two of us remembering our stride in unison before we left. For a brief moment, my wings broke through my shoulder blades and I was a runner anticipating the sound of the gunfire to begin racing the wind. My brain wasn't swimming and my body wasn't bracing for impact. For a half of a second, I felt alive for the first time since dare I whisper yet again, our before. But I was dead, living amongst the barely alive, and the slide to our inevitable death was all uphill. It is beyond sick and twisted that we cannot appreciate the truest value of life until we are face-to-face with death. The turmoil of the inner tug of war was both daunting and invigorating, my cheerleader and my nemesis. Even out in the world, I couldn't find my footing. There was such a vast space, yet I did not fit. There was only one space that suited my tattered edges and I was currently far too far from her. I had to go back. The irony was there was no going back, but there was no moving forward either. All that existed in our world was the present. All we had was our now. We lived both in the here and the there but truly nowhere. We were a dead version of the living, attempting to stay alive. We took up space both in our world and in theirs, finding our place in between the in-between. The walk had taken up too much precious time that I didn't have to spare and my claustrophobic thoughts were catapulting me down a spiral. Chief guided me back to our in-between. I found my home in the place that knows no space - her.

The following day, we celebrated her eight-month milestone as if it were her first birthday. Facing death forces you to wish on candles every day. The rise and fall of her chest was like a chocolate world to me. Her every breath was celebrated as only one being knows how many breaths she will take. I sat on the porch swing with her cradled in my arms, clinging desperately to every breath that kissed my skin. The soon-to-be summer breeze was showing off, performing a private contemporary dance just for us. These brief moments were the rope we clung to, like a screen door swimming in the core of a tsunami. The little things were our small victories amongst the endless losses. It was a constant tug of war between the never ending to do lists and the savoring of every moment as if it were our last, because it very well could have been. We had tasted the tasteless and more cardboard was on the way. Bath time turned into wrinkled skin as every drop of heat was soaked in. Watching her smile at the delight of soapy bubbles was worth every minute that ticked by. My gaze was blackened by the hauntings up ahead, as I knew all too well what was coming. I longed for nothing more than just to stay right there, in the now cold bubble bath. Smiling through gritted teeth, pretending it was and would all be okay, praying desperately in my head that we'd make it. I would make every attempt to find sunshine and rainbows despite being constantly blanketed in storm clouds and a darkness that made my blood run cold. Before diagnosis, I had plans for her first birthday. Since diagnosis, I only prayed we'd make it through the night and be gifted with the rise of the morn. I found an endless gratitude for today, knowing that tomorrow may never come.

Tomorrow came and I had scheduled a family photo shoot. Not to memorialize the nightmare that had become our life, but to bask in the gift of life we had been given. I adored my skin and bones with a dress that hung on me. I dressed her in baby blues that held no competition for her eyes and attempted to look beyond her steroid-ridden face. It was chaotic and complicated, but beautiful nonetheless. We smiled through the thoughts that these may be our last family photos together. There was nothing fake about our grins. In fact, we had never been more real. With the busy of the day, she fell asleep on my chest and I couldn't help but hope that when she finds age 25, she'll still be falling asleep on me. The bliss of the moment was wiped out by black hollow images that stood before me feeding on my soul. The next day we would go in for counts and I hated this eve. My skin became clammy and cold, making a reptile look like a coat of fur. A lump grew in my throat the size of a basketball, making it impossible to swallow and I shoved down the vomit that longed to escape. The pit of my stomach caressed my spine, leaving me feeling empty and full at the same time. My atrophied muscle was unable to move as it was paralyzed with fear. My breath was labored while my chest antagonistically threatened to cave in. I was bathing in his darkness, desperately clinging to my maker's light. As my claws chipped away at the dirt, I begged God to pull us in. Not close enough to bring us home, but to grant us a stay here together, a boat far away from the dark angel's grip. But who was I to dictate? I am but a selfish human. There I lay with his deathly breath on my neck causing every hair to stand in formation. I was like a fire ant scaling the walls of a cave with a waterfall pouring in. I focused my sight on the smidgen of light in the far-off distance, seen by some miracle through squinted eyes. While being consumed by the dark shadows, I bargained my losses for her win.

I lost myself to the devil in the night, but God granted her a win in the morning. She made counts. We were able to soak home in for one more night as the following day we would be back in the ring. The house smelled of a home-cooked meal and kept me from falling too far down the rabbit hole while I packed for the unknown. I soaked our pillows, holding onto her as we laid together in gratitude, hoping for many nights like this in the someday. The night was everlasting and the morning all too quick, but with war paint on our faces and boxing gloves on our hands, we re-entered the battlefield. Immediately, tubes and wires bound us to the bed. She screamed out in protest as she was hungry, but I was not allowed to feed her. The irony was she had developed an aversion to food. She feared every object that came within a five-mile radius of her mouth as it would cause her pain. The dance parties, cheerleading and confetti thrown in attempts to help her embrace her human instinct to eat were completely negated by moments such as this. Any time she had to go under anesthesia, she had to be NPO, which means nothing by mouth. This would begin at midnight the night prior and lasted until after she awoke from anesthesia the following day. Hunger was not the issue, but the confusion of either being denied food or being fearful of pain created a devastating setback in her relationship with food.

I pulled her in as if my hug would soothe the growls in her belly. We walked down endless morgue-like hallways. Strangers longed to touch her, but their touch alone could take her which only caused me to pull her in even closer. There was always so much waiting which birthed hauntings of reliving moments I wish I could forget. The tears, like waterfalls, bathed my face as I pulled on every ear in the room speaking only with my eyes. I whispered as loud as I could, beckoning her ear drum. I told her to keep breathing. No matter what, she had to keep breathing. There was no time for turning purple and no room for the PICU. I told her over and over again to just breathe. I told her to come back to me and that they would take care of her. I told her I would be right here and to just keep breathing. I was clutching her like a thief with his riches, resisting every encouragement that pushed me to let her go. Every one of their eyes were on me, urging me to put my hands up. I would have rather died than let her go, but holding onto her meant she could die. After lathering her in my kisses and tears, I unwillingly handed her over, begging them to bring her back to me. Their backs turned to face me and my gaze never left the crown of her tiny head. When the doors closed, I was emptier than a hollowed-out barrel rotting in a southern swamp. I sat in a chair sprinkled with germs, pager and phone in hand. I waited in a crowded room with city-like noise. I hate the city and the chaos was deafening. All I could hear was her cry and my mind daydreamed of her sweet face. Every inch of me wanted to run back through those doors and find my way back to her. But I followed the rules, stayed seated, tapped my feet on the sticky floor distracting myself from my insanity. I summoned my thoughts to telepathically make their way to her, "Keep breathing Dakota Ann, do you hear Mama? Breathe."

My name called out, drowning out the sounds of the torture chamber. My heart sank to the heels of my feet and my stomach twisted like a wrung-out rag with not one drop left. I ran as fast as I could to the desk, but my feet felt like they were 30 yards behind me. The receptionist smiled and I wondered how she could find a smile in a dungeon such as this, blissfully unaware. I was more than prepared to sprint through the doors, but she met my excitement with defeat, informing me that they were done and I could go back shortly. Like a first grader, I couldn't help but ask exactly how long "shortly" was. Her smile was crooked and I noticed her hesitant mannerisms. I shamefully made my way back to my seat. Shortly came way too long after and was followed by more hallways leading to hell's gates. It was like a mad maze in a haunted house where clowns mock your cries. I hate clowns. I saw her bird cage and I felt like I was sprinting, but I was at a standstill. My baby was swollen, red and teasing lifelessness, but her chest moved. I slapped my own hands at my every instinct to reach through the bars that divided us. I was not allowed to hold her, but my eyes scanned every inch of her. She was pale with swirls of red, ballooned and taut. Her skin looked as if it had been held captive by flames but its touch burned like ice. I wanted to crawl into the darkest corner of the room, find the fetal position and beg for death. I stood with every bit of strength I could summon, whispering, "Mama is here." Her eyes began to move and I called her back with desperation in my voice. It took what felt like an eternity, but she came to. Her cry was that of a 50-year chain smoker. My hands were sweating while my fingers pill rolled to keep me from a forbidden embrace. I reminded myself to wait despite my every inclination to grab her and run. This was worse than being suspended from the ceiling with my insides being removed piece by piece. Minutes ticked by like centuries, and my impatience consumed the room. A calmness blanketed us all once she was in my arms.

Through the webbing of tubes and wires, being sure not to rip anything embedded inside her, we were both home. She was wailing and red with fury. She would calm in doses and then release her agony, rinse, repeat. The nurse asked if I wanted her to take her. I can't imagine what my eyes said, but my mouth let out an assertive *no*. I loathed this version of me I had become. We both found peace intertwined in one another. I was placed in a wheelchair with her in my lap, rollercoasting our way back upstairs. She slept for a short while but, awoke in an even more escalated state. I was breaking eardrums and cracking walls in attempts to get someone to see that something was wrong. She was climbing up my torso as if snakes and wolves were waiting, mouths open wide below. Nothing was easing her pain. Her ears were like fire, her face round, purple and lathered in tears. Her team offered pain medication. Just the word alone was like swallowing down bleach, but I wouldn't make the same mistake twice. They tried Tylenol first which helped her to find sleep, but she would let out these soft sobs even in her rest. With every whimper, my mama heart was like a broken mirror shattered on the floor. Her team then suggested morphine. I envisioned broken souls in dark alleyways swaying in the strobe lights of the city, begging the night to end it all. My infant was a broken soul, enduring a darkness I couldn't begin to fathom. There was no swaying as she could barely hold her head up. There were no lights, only shadows of the creatures playing hot potato with her life. She was pleading with the night and begging me to make it stop. She received morphine.

CHAPTER 3

$\mathcal{M}$orphine perked her up at first. She laughed and smiled while her head rolled around on her shoulders. She eventually found a sound sleep and despite my heart being broken at the thought of morphine, it was at peace with her peace. She awoke with a smile and I gave her a smile back - my girl. Just as we began to find light, the curtains were drawn and the 24-hour chemo started. It came again, like a bat out of hell. The back of her head fell between her shoulder blades. A cry escaped her body like that of a demon that had been locked away for decades. Her skin was ablaze, fire roasted and hot out of the oven. She was climbing me like a tree trunk, wrapping herself around my head, terrified of the hands grasping for her below. This episode came at a lightning speed and faded just as quickly. She found her daddy's chest and they hummed together. They sang a song only the two of them understood. It was a heartbreaking whale cry of loss and loneliness, but somehow soothing and disgustingly beautiful. She found sleep buried in his chest, but it was short lived and within 30 minutes, she was challenging the night's silence with what was left of her voice box. Her cries tore through every heart in the room, leaving tattered pieces that were once whole in her wave of destruction. She was refusing to drink and swatting away anything that remotely touched her skin as if touch were branding her. She pushed down hard through her belly, almost as if to expel from deep within, but she was empty, leaving nothing but excruciating pain. We gave her more morphine, which landed her back in Daddy's arms, exhausted but comfortable. Morphine would make her nose itch and did not completely eliminate her pain, but it provided a tolerance and relief to an extent. Morphine allowed her sleep despite making my skin birth an army of tarantulas. Morphine. My infant was on morphine.

There were so many drugs, yet not enough. Methotrexate is a strong chemotherapy drug that can cause chemical-like burns both inside and outside of the body. This drug would run through Dakota over a 24-hour period. She had a catheter placed to decrease the output coming into contact with her skin in hopes to prevent burns. After the 24 hours, she would have to clear it through urine output. She was placed on fluids to help run it out of her system more quickly. This increased her output which increased her risk of burns. Changing a dirty diaper with a catheter and toxic waste is not a task any motherhood book prepares anyone for. It was poison coming out of all ends. She would dry heave several times, causing this smoker-like cough to coat the back of her throat. Then projectile vomit would come and keep coming, like an exorcist but chemical fumes would arise from the secretions. After over 72 hours of dousing her in morphine and methotrexate like holy water, we were granted a trip away from our padded room.

They were like dueling rivers, methotrexate and morphine, flowing effortlessly through my infant daughter's veins. One scorching her from the inside and the other feeding the flames. Her bi-polar state was telling the story playing out inside her. One minute, she was playing and reading books. The next, like she was being doused in gasoline surrounded by lit matches. It was as if we were in a cage hanging just above the lava coursing through the valleys of death. The bubbles would burst and splash our flesh, like acid melting us through bone. There was an untouchable agony that taunted the heart to cease the beat of its drum, a helplessness that leaves suicide the only plate on the table. No matter what room we were in, we were still seduced by the evil of the night. We were becoming zombies, eternally numb from enduring a pain made not just for death, but extinction. We were drained of every drop of humanness we had left. In a hail Mary to keep our hearts beating, we were granted a trip home, without morphine and off of methotrexate. Another hail Mary was thrown our way when the phone rang with light on the other end. She was now MRD (minimal residual disease) negative, clinical remission. Forget the dam. We embodied the entire ocean. Like life had been breathed into our lungs, we came alive. We were dead humans resuscitated by the venom of a vampire, died and reborn. The adrenaline rush birthed a superhuman strength to push back on the rivers. The war of good verses evil was alive in the wake of death, but love was still winning. We still had a pulse.

Even in the in-between, she was struggling through her battle. She refused to eat, but would drink in small increments. She was fighting through nausea, vomiting and diarrhea. I was giving her medications to help through a syringe. Morning and night, I was swinging, but everything I attempted to put in was coming right out. During one of her vomiting episodes, we found a lesion under her tongue that bought us a trip to the ER. Everything is possibly something and nothing is ever nothing in the pediatric cancer world. The lesion was an injury from a previous intubation and was showing signs of healing. We were able to go back to the in-between for further healing until we were readmitted to the battlefield. She began sleeping much more than her normal, which wasn't saying much as sleep was not her friend. The dry heaving that turned into violent vomiting worsened and we were admitted early due to mucositis. Her mouth was covered in cauliflower heads causing blood and saliva to pour out of her mouth. What we could visibly see was more than likely barely scratching the surface of the hell scene raging inside her. She was being treated for nausea, dehydration and pain in hopes of making her body as strong as physically possible for the beating she would begin to endure in the morning. We were stuck on repeat in a horror film, where the monster just keeps coming without tiring, and the places to hide were slimming. We were desperate to stop, to give her a chance to heal, but a chance at healing would leave the door wide open for cancer to score a goal. We were on a vertical mudslide in flip flops and the next wave was hell bent on wiping us out.

There's no place like home, there's no place like home, there was no home. Twenty-four-hour chemo began. She was screaming and choking. Blood and saliva were pouring from her lips, pooling in the back of her throat. White blisters coated her from one end to the other like poison ivy. I held her close, both of us drenched in sweat. I bounced her, sang lullabies, sobbed in the interim and prayed with desperation, begging Him to hear our cries. She fell asleep from pure exhaustion and I placed her down in the cage. But no move was the right move and she woke with vengeance. She was gurgling like a clogged drain beckoning from a sink. I picked her up, placing her in her spot on me as she dry heaved violently over my left shoulder. She threw herself back and squeezed her shoulder blades together as if a demon had taken over her infant body. There was not a prayer left in my sails. I was more defeated than that of a marathoner who didn't cross the finish line, watching the men pack up red sashes and archways. With my own head falling between my shoulder blades, I told her, "I'm trying baby, I am trying so hard." She curled her shoulders forward and projectile vomited. I gave her Zofran, an anti-nausea medication. We were all well beyond nausea. Her legs gave out and she finally succumbed to the feat of the marathon.

I laid her down and threw in the towel myself. What felt like seconds later, like a priest was waterboarding her in holy water, the exorcism began again. They gave her IV Benadryl and morphine in attempts to help her through the storm. She immediately started convulsing. I said, "She's seizing! She's seizing!"

One of the 25 voices in the room said, "No her eyes are tracking. It's not a seizure." She couldn't stop flailing. Her whole body was thrashing like a baby bird making every attempt not to fall to its death. The room quickly grew claustrophobic, packed to the brim with bodies, flashlights, stethoscopes and over 100 different opinions. I begged from the bottom of my desperate mama heart for immediate answers. It was like watching her drown just a few feet in front of me, but I was entangled in metal chains. Suddenly, like a heavenly wave, the episode subsided. Her shoulder blades returned to neutral, her head found a happy medium and she wasn't attempting to fly away. But her legs were still stuck out to sea treading water, trying to stay above the surface. Her belly contracted, locked and loaded. She opened her mouth and the demon released. There were bodies on hands and knees, sopping up the blood and poison, gloved and masked to be sure not to inhale death themselves.

I was still standing with her in my arms attempting to "it's okay" the "not okay". I felt a warm wetness touch my stomach. She was wet. We were both wet, which only meant that her catheter was no longer working. The toxins were bathing our skin and like acid, she was melting. The chaos consumed the revolving door and I took less than five seconds to lose myself in the bathroom in order to push through the barricades up ahead. When I came out, the room was empty, but I could hear her screaming. I followed the sound of her cries and found another room across the hall. I let myself in, unaware of the forever nightmare I was entering. The lights were so bright they were blinding. There was a buzzing so loud it made my eyes squint. Three nurses were holding her down and she was making the all too white paint crack at the pitch of her screams. I ran to her side, again whispering "okays" in the "nowhere near okay".

Her catheter had completely come out so they were attempting to place it back in. They pushed inside of her and she let out a sound that sliced my breath. One of the nurses said, "There's resistance." I fixed my eyes on her hair line being sure not to fray a strand with my fireballs. I couldn't help but think, *of course there is resistance*. They were attempting to shove something inside her, a place inside her that should know no shoving of any kind. They pushed again and she tied the score with her protest. They pushed. She resisted. They pushed harder and her body slid up the table as all remaining human pieces of me died an excruciating death. They pushed again and despite her intense effort, they won. It was in.

The walls were shattering at the sound of her cries. She had torn everything down beyond the studs. We made our way back to our room, like a victim walks the street after a gruesome attack. We all walked a walk of shame that to this very day haunts our attempts at dreams. She was wired, like an addict tweaking. She was rubbing her eyes but she was wide awake. Her eyes were bulging out of her head. Her body was twitching uncontrollably. She was as high as a kite, yet like a rolling boil inside. I was bouncing her, rocking her, trying so damn hard to make it better in the battle uphill. An hour and a half later she gave in and I placed her back in the cage hoping for a drop of rest. I closed my eyes for one half of a second only to be awakened by her vomiting. Teams of people began piling in. We sat her up to help let it all escape. More gloved hands filled with towels, cleaning up a mixture of blood and toxic bile. I pulled her in close and the wet warmth returned on my skin. I tossed my head back in defeat, as my legs struggled to hold us both in standing. The catheter wasn't working again and we had not an ounce of strength to press rewind on the scene we had just barely made it through less than an hour ago. After much debate, they took it out and left it out. I guess in some sick sense, you could call that a win. She was inconsolable and the vomiting had an everlasting battery. We gave her more morphine. We hadn't yet slept, but the morning had come. They performed a weight check and blood draw. I continued bouncing, rocking, trying to keep us both alive. She continued vomiting. They continued cleaning. I made an attempt at words, but I had killed my voice with my screams. I wouldn't put her down. I was terrified to let her go, in every way. We built a U-shape at the top of her bed to allow the secretions to slide out of the corner of her mouth, in hopes of keeping her from drowning in her own toxin-filled fluids. I gently let her body fall away from mine as I watched blood pour from her lips. She started to grind her teeth to ease the pain. It is said that there is no pain like watching your child know pain and yet there is nothing you can do to stop their pain. Pain is a butterfly tasting the sweet nectar from a pink flower on a Spring day in May. There are no human words for this kind of pain.

We gave her more morphine for her pain. I sat on that couch, drowning in a pain that no pain medication could touch. I was more alone than that of a message in a bottle drifting in the middle of the ocean. Barely holding onto faith as we were being tossed to the roof of the devil's mouth like an orca playing with a seal, splashing onto his serpent tongue. Like a wounded soldier with his face in the mud, the blood of his brother on his lips and the dirt of his enemy's boot in his teeth, I looked up to watch her chest. Intently, I watched it rise and fall, but it rose again. I scrolled through the contacts in my phone. Everyone says, "If you need anything, just call." But I didn't know a soul on this earth who could possibly comprehend the words that I couldn't speak. My screams were deafening, yet I was mute. I was grateful for the bracelets, the orange rocks, and all of the support. I saw their touch without them physically being with me, but I was fearful of touching them back. I was beyond death, but never more alive. I had died over and over again, but I wasn't living a life. I didn't click on anyone's name because I didn't want to intrude. I didn't want to wake them from their dreams and spill over my nightmares. I didn't want them to know what I had known. I wanted to protect them from the hell I had seen. I shut off my phone and sat more alone in my darkness. I allowed it to take me, like watching the surface fade as the anchor pulled me to the ocean's floor. I didn't fight as I had no fight left. I swallowed down the bitterness of the agony and tasted the sweetness of death. Again.

The days and nights began to blend together into one. As I picked her up, I felt it immediately. Under her arm pits was like hot bath water. I pushed the red button, beckoning the cross for the hundredth time in the last hour. I told them she was warm and I was almost certain she had a fever. Mama knows. They took her temperature and sure enough, it was 100.9. Fevers meant infections and infections could take her away. My heart began drumming outside of my chest. Her heat increased and with its rise, my stomach twisted like the thread in the needle knitting the most intricate quilt. The needle moving in and out, up and down, through and through. Worst rollercoaster ever.

A few nurses flowed in, adorned in gowns and masks. They placed her on three different types of antibiotics and ran blood cultures to test for infections. Vitals were done in sequence as per usual. Temperature, blood pressure, pulse ox and overall appearance. The wiring was placed after, two on her chest and two on her back. More monitors. The room was unusually quiet as our tongues were tied and our hearts were broken. We sat on the couch watching the chaos, completely helpless. Blood pressures were always exhausting as she would scream and kick when the cuff began to tighten, only making the numbers climb.

My instinct was to bounce, sway and coo it all away, but we both had to remain still and quiet in hopes of a satisfactory reading. Unsatisfactory meant we had to stop and start again. Again, again, again and again. We both ended up drenched, panting and longing for a five second break before the next test began.

At the conclusion of a series of tests for all of 10 minutes, my hands found her body through the wiring and pulled her in close. One of the antibiotics ran for 30 minutes, then a flush. Another ran for an hour, then another flush. The last one ran for an hour, followed by one more flush. By the end, she wouldn't drink as she was choking on her own saliva and blood. Her right eye was barely open due to the number of fluids she was receiving to help her body flush out the methotrexate. I attempted to give her the oral medications, but she started choking. With her in my arms and 12 pairs of eyes on us, I couldn't help but panic. She had to take in the medications, but she couldn't swallow them down. My once strong shoulders were a wet blanket pooling at my feet. They suggested more morphine in hopes of helping her swallow her medications as they are not available intravenously. The morphine helped her to swallow down a little at a time. She drifted off, but awoke worse than before. Her fever had returned. Her nose began to bleed. I attempted to give her Tylenol orally, but she threw it up immediately. She was screaming and I was a blubbering mess. My husband was trying to hold us both up. Both of us were saying, "It's okay, it's okay." But none of this was okay. This was not okay. We were not okay, but we had no other option than to be, okay.

It was decided around five that evening, that a morphine drip would be best to help manage her pain. What was less than okay was an infant on a morphine drip. It was set to give her a scheduled dose around the clock, but I was instructed to push a button if I felt she needed more. No pressure. It allotted me to push in 15-minute increments. She was chewing on my shirt and grinding her teeth. It was like nails on a chalkboard causing my insides to cringe. She was enduring such an enormity of pain that she had to physically bite down and grind her teeth in order to distract herself from the agony. The sound of her teeth coursing against each other echoed through my eardrum. I am her mother and my sole purpose is to make it better. The button beckoned me just beneath my fingertips. Her grinding was like a devilish cackle teasing me like a school girl on an elementary playground. I knew the parameters were set according to mathematical logic, but I feared the effects of such a powerful drug on her tiny body. I was involuntarily playing the most horrific game of tug of war, and there was no winning. I gently wiped the blood, spit, blisters and chemo away. I wiped so tenderly, being sure not to rip open any more parts of her that were already exposed. She let out a scream that cut me so deeply my flesh has yet to recover. I pushed the button. She began coughing and the she couldn't stop. She was fully submerged in an uncontrollable coughing fit, drowning in her own secretions. Meanwhile, I was waterboarding myself with mom guilt. I was wracking my brain, attempting to decipher if it was the mucositis inhibiting her ability to swallow, or the downward push of my thumb suppressing her respiratory system. I could hear the cement hardening in her lungs as she dug deeper to clear her throat. I watched the clock like a soldier on night watch, anxiously waiting in the space between the 15 minutes. With my eyes closed in shame and my brows frowning towards my nose, I pushed again. I pulled her in closer, not that there were any gaps between us that could be sealed. We searched the night sky through the hospital blinds, silently begging for a sign of light in our dark.

It must have just struck around nine because I heard fireworks. But our world was so immensely dark we couldn't see them, no sense in the tease anyway. I imagined families sitting on threaded blankets in tall grass looking up at the colors painting the sky. I envisioned their smile, soaking in such a simple pleasure of a summer night in July. I was envious and jealous, yet hopeful for someday, maybe. Her cheek kissed mine and I whispered softly in her ear, "You hold on, you hear me? I know it hurts but you hold on." She responded with a whimper that let me know she was barely holding on, so I pushed. I rocked her and told her it would be okay but none of this was okay. Would it ever be okay? She fell asleep with her head buried in my chest but awoke within minutes screaming and choking. Blood and saliva, thick as tar, poured from lips. I pushed. She reached for my face as if to tell me, "It's okay." The guilt gutted me and I bled out on the tile floor feeling so unworthy of her love. I kissed her poor cheeks that were red and angry like they had been burnt by the sun. She was melting from the inside out from the very thing that was meant to save her life, yet it was taking her physically. I pushed.

Daddy and I were engulfed in our own fire, fueled by an anger that had an untouchable depth. We bit down hard, fighting back the words we wouldn't be able to take back and pushing hard on the dam. She was beyond exhausted but her body couldn't rest. Her screams were stripping the paint from the walls. It took every ounce of strength we had left to not match her screams with our own. I pushed. Around midnight, we embodied a smushed pumpkin and the attending suggested that maybe the lights from her sound machine or the crib were making her upset. I made every attempt to remain human and not chew her face off with my mama bear teeth. We had been living in the hospital for months on end. The blood curdling noises releasing from her body had absolutely nothing to do with her sound machine or the bird cage. Her pain was coming from the demons torturing her in unison inside her, leaving us all to throw question marks and eurekas at the wall at what we couldn't see. I gave her an *A* for effort despite my eyes meeting the back of my head and I pushed. She suggested Ativan so we made a swing and missed. I pushed.

She was suffering and our tools were depleted. Everything we threw at the wall bounced off and met our foreheads with mockery. We were literally screaming and although we were heard, we were unheard. Like taking an evening stroll after the moon has risen and walking by a house with walls vibrating from the sounds. You want to look down and pretend your ears aren't ringing from the volume. Part of you is curiously concerned, but the polite human in you pushes your feet forward in your walk. We dulled our voices at the sound of footsteps to decrease the casualties in our octagon, but deep down we were desperate for someone to save us from our blows. The three of us were breaking in ways we didn't know were humanly possible. She was being destroyed physically while we were enduring psychotic breaks from the emotional anguish in failing at our one job: shielding her from pain. She was making sounds that will forever haunt my daydreams, a wheeze that gasped for air like two lone fingers clutching the side of a cliff. The night swallowed each one of us whole and by the cusp of morning, we had no fight left. We had laid down our swords and accepted our defeat. The darkness had won.

With the sun's rise, she was still in my arms. I was still bouncing and rocking. My arms were so numb, I barely felt the weight. In fast forward and in slow motion, her head fell away from my left shoulder. Her skin turned an awful shade of gray, her lips a deep purple, and her eyes rolled back in her head. My mind was shouting the one word my tongue couldn't speak: *dead*. I was holding her in my arms assuming her death before my eyes. I swore she was gone. I was searching her lifeless body for light, but I only imagined her angel wings above me. I longed for death so immensely. I felt what pieces of life I had left from the night before fall to their death at my feet, and I embraced it like a tall glass of water in the Arizona heat. I started screaming at the top of my lungs, "She's not breathing!!! HELP!!! PLEASE HELP!!! She's not breathing!!!!!" He had caught us with our guard down and took the fatal swing. It was assisted murder, his swinging combined with my pushing caused her death. I took away her breath and since, I have never allowed myself to inhale.

An angel in blue came rushing into our room. She heard my screams. She immediately scooped Dakota in her arms and started blowing in her face. The seconds that ticked by all too slowly felt like years. I pleaded, "Please Dakota come back." Her body startled but went limp again. Before I could blink, over 10 people began filling the room. Like a windshield in a torrential downpour, I could barely see through my tears. They placed her in her crib and began suctioning. I begged again, "God please, please don't take my baby. Please Lord, please don't take my baby." I called to her, "Dakota I am right here, please come back baby. Come on baby, breathe please!" I was sandwiched between two of her doctors and they were both insisting that she would be okay. Their mouths were speaking words that their eyes clearly did not have full faith in, but they were great at their job, assuring me it would be okay in the not okay. I physically felt hands on my back, but like a corpse I felt nothing as I was dead inside. I cried out to the chaos of the room, "Please save my baby." She was eerily quiet and her silence deafened the madness of the room. A pause button stuck in place. Time was moving forward but our scene remained at a standstill. Like a switch, her cheeks began to look flushed. I've never been happier to see lobster cheeks. She screamed and I am certain even non-believers let out a hallelujah.

How sweet the sound, I was screaming from 10 feet away; "I'm right here Dakota. Mama is right here." Her crib was surrounded by more bodies than I could count. I've never been in a stock room, but I imagine this room takes the cake. They placed a tube that looked like a pool noodle in comparison to her tiny body, down her throat. It was louder than 10 vacuums and more powerful too as it pulled out tar-like blood along with a yellow translucent glue from deep inside her chest. It was abundant and filled 10 ounces of a cup that hung inconspicuously on the wall behind her crib. Ten ounces of secretions. She was drowning. "I'm so sorry Dakota." The molasses was endless, like a river with no destination. Her screams grew louder and louder as her voice was being freed of its suppressions. Faces I knew all too well entered the room with looks of fear and defeat. I usually felt better when I saw those faces but on this particular battlefield, they resembled lost soldiers. Their eyes spoke volumes despite their mouths not uttering a sound. My heart sank to a depth beyond this world and my blood lost every ounce of warmth. The cold rush blanketed me as I tasted the smell of the morgue.

With our forever drawers side-by-side, they began throwing hail Mary's while performing chest X-rays. I was asked to go out into the hall in order to safely perform the imaging. With my jaw on the floor and my feet cemented into the tile, I couldn't leave her. I had just lived out the worst-case scenario, my child's death. And now I was being asked to separate our space and breathe different air. The only thought I could muster was, *over my dead body*, but I was in fact already dead. I waited out in the hall with the army that was attempting to keep her here. I paced and updated my husband with words I couldn't believe I was saying. Her chest X-rays were clear and it was time to pack as we were headed to PICU. Like soldiers, we piled back into her room. She was pale, yet marbled with purple like that of a grape on its way out. My eyes found the faces I trusted most and without a word spoken, I made it known that leaving them was the last thing I wanted to do. They placed a mask over Dakota's broken face to help her find breath. Our angel brought Dakota to me to hold her for the first time since I let her go. I felt undeserving, a shame that has never left me. She was warm, pink and breathing. *Keep breathing, please.* I searched her face for I was drowning as she was swimming her way to the surface. I thought she was gone. I truly thought I had lost her. My very worst nightmare had come true. My baby girl had died. But she was still here, in my arms. I could see her, feel her warmth, and witness the rise and fall of her chest. She was colorless and dead. Now she was too beautifully red and alive. My brain couldn't compute the spectrum of extremes and my heart was still slicing me with shards of glass created by guilt. I have always been unworthy of her, but from here on out, I would forever be worth less. She had died and I was left to endure the agony of her loss at my hand. She was alive and I was now living out my own self-inflicted death. I had to place her back in the birdcage to be transferred down to the PICU. The holding her, then letting her go, both physically and metaphorically, was a mind game that created open wounds unable to develop scars. I marched beside her angels as we walked her down to the dungeon. Like the men that carry the coffin up the aisle in church, except she was still alive.

Similar to the transition between the church and the cemetery, the air changed immediately and we were suffocated by the bitterness of the PICU. Encased in liquid nitrogen, the scars from our burns during our prior stay surfaced. Walking down hallways far louder than a summer carnival, yet they embody the silence of a wake. The rules are four people in the room at a time, yet there was an overflow of people spilling out of this one room. Like driving slowly past the ambulance, you can't help but look at the flashing lights. A father hovered over his baby girl, sobbing. Her body was only slightly bigger than my own baby girl. She was adorned in the same diaper, wiring and tubing. My heart hugged her daddy from the hallway as we walked by. We arrived at our room in the basement with barely a sliver of a window. To my surprise, a friendly face arrived. She smiled unlike the other faces. There were towers of machines placed on both sides of Dakota's birdcage. Doubled beeping means double the insanity. She looked as if she had just escaped the gates of hell and I have no doubt she did. I couldn't help but beat the crap out of myself with a metal bat that screamed with every hit, "You did this!"

I pushed, over and over and over again. I never pushed outside of the 15-minute increments, but my pushing within the parameters assisted in stealing her breath. *I'm so sorry*. She was already drowning and in my failed attempts to decrease her pain, I held her head under the water. I have carried dark ghosts with me my entire life, but this heavy hitter takes the cake and leaves a trail. I didn't want to take my eyes off of her, yet I couldn't look her in the eye. I damn near killed her and my head, buried in quicksand, wouldn't be enough to hold shame. She had open blisters lathered throughout her inner tubing making it incredibly painful to clear the secretions. Therefore, all of the fluid, the blood, the saliva and the mucous pooled in her airway. The longer it sat there, the thicker and more solidified it became, making the already difficult to clear all the more difficult to clear. The perfect storm of her inability to keep her airway open in conjunction with my incessant pushing became lethal and damn near fatal. Or maybe this is just what they told me to keep me from taking my own life as I almost took her life. I gave another *A* for their efforts and I will never not want to strip myself of my own breath for taking her breath. Oxygen now provided her breath. She was blanketed in everything meant to help keep her alive and shielded from my touch that could take her breath. Her chemo had cleared from her body so they stopped her fluids, but her body then revolted and spiked a fever. A fever meant infection and an infection meant possible death. Hadn't we faced enough death in the last few hours? She needed Tylenol, but they only had it in a liquid form requiring it to be taken orally. She had just endured a near drowning experience due to the inability to swallow and now we were to force her to choke down medication in hopes of not losing her due to a fever. If there was ever a question as to the padded room we will forever live in, revert back to this day alone. The nurse with the smile face helped us help her to fight through the gurgles of purple slime that oozed out of the corner of her mouth. I scooped the purple goop off of her burnt skin and as gently as I possibly could, I placed it back in her mouth, begging her to swallow it down. The look she gave me is one that stole my rights as a mother with but one glance. I knew she was in agony and swallowing was the source, yet I was forcing her to gulp down, inflicting her pain once again with my own hand. I have been told time and time again that she will never remember any of this, but I myself will never forget.

I stood on a stool at her bedside, reliving every disgraceful scene of the night before, for every ear in the room to hear. The barely out of high school looking doctor apologized so hard in his grin, I couldn't help but believe him. But I knew the truth more than I could humanly bear and the sound of my own voice giving the play by play was pushing me dangerously close to the edge. With my child size pinky toe barely gripping the ledge, I yelled out, "I did it okay!!! I almost killed my daughter!!" No truer words were spoken and there was nothing left to say. We had beaten the hell out of all of the words, but he continued to speak, attempting to convince me otherwise. Their efforts were commendable. Eventually, exhaustion overpowered the voices in the room. She had finally found rest for the first time in well over 24 hours and it was time to put down our microphones. She was still breathing and the losses had to be put to bed for another day. We were under PICU rules, therefore only one of us could be in the room with her for sleep. My husband had no energy to find a room to sleep in, so he slept in his car. Our daughter just died in my arms and now we had to increase the distance between us as if there wasn't already enough.

I was alone with her and I didn't feel I should have been permitted to be alone with her. I did just play Russian roulette with her life. I remained close enough to where she could feel my love, but I stayed far enough away to be sure not to hurt her anymore. She looked defeated, like an Ironman still a couple of yards from the finish line. He could see the red sash, but his body was barely moving. His legs like rooted trunks and his feet encased in cement struggling to stay upright. With barely a drop left of air in his lungs, and the ground beneath him begging him to lay down. I couldn't help but ask myself if she was done. Was her body too tired? At what point is enough, enough? I longed for her to find the words to tell me where she stood. I wanted her voice to give me the physical beating I so well deserved. I was desperate to give her exactly what she needed and wanted as I was incapable of making those decisions for her. But her less than one-year-old mind could not create the words to describe the insanity of the most recent events, let alone comprehend them. I, once a person of a sound mind, had neither the words nor the understanding of this version of hell either.

With her body still ablaze, she would sleep for 30 minutes at a time. It was a restless rest. My eyes never found the back of my head as I was determined to not allow the night to take us captive again. With the rise of the sun, her oxygen was lowered. She had even more mucositis, as if her body hadn't had enough open cauliflower heads spreading inside of her. Her sucking thumb looked like an angry demon - red, swollen and blistered. There was barely an inch of her flesh that wasn't scorched from the most recent wildfire. She had no fever or infections, which in and of itself was a win, and she was breathing without oxygen. Her face was mangled. Her flesh was exposed like wide open curtains. Her gasping for air was showcased on her face and the adhesive from the tape was a fresh flame to her sensitive chemo skin. She was worn, a fighter in the 10th round, with another round on deck. She was huddled in the corner with sweat dripping from her brow, spitting blood in the ring. Her eyes had darkened by a shade and she could barely hold her head up, but she was still breathing. *Keep breathing, Dakota Ann.*

With breath in her lungs, I felt safe enough to go use the ladies' room although my score card showed my red flags, so I am not so sure any of my choices could be deemed safe. I walked out of our room and down the hall. There were so many people in this one room still. There were even more bodies spilling onto the floor. I was baffled by the rules and even in my wrecked state, I was able to compute that this could only mean one thing. The infant fighter was face down in the ring with the ref too close to counting her out.

That feeling of life being drained from your body all at once washed over me and my heart sank to a new depth. That feeling was becoming all too normal for me. I walked through another set of doors, only to find more people flooding the space that had no space. Some were standing against the wall. Nurses were sitting on the cold tile, and grown men were holding one another up. I couldn't help but overhear one man saying to another, "She's going to a better place. She won't suffer anymore." Like a sledgehammer to a mirror, I shattered in unison with them. I walked outside gasping for air and ironically, it was a beautiful night. A blue sky painted with pale pinks and purples, splashes of bright orange. The wind was enough for a strong kiss, but not enough to romance you off of your feet. Perfection. Looking back at the brick walls, knowing what was happening behind those closed doors, I became engulfed with fury. I was spiraling down a rabbit hole in confusion. I demanded He explain. I screamed at the sky, begging Him to tell me why. Why did my baby find breath again, but this baby was taking her last? Why?

I was drowning in the inner turmoil of guilt. I had anchors on my feet, treading water in a hurricane. I was trapped by a circle made of oil and lit ablaze. Dakota was on the sinking ship 30 feet in front of me and the other baby was less than a foot away being taunted by a pack of tiger sharks. I yelled to Him, "It's not a tradeoff and it shouldn't be!" I know in my right mind that that is not the way it works, but in my fit of desperation and rage, the gang-like deal seemed far too real for me. I was antagonized by His beauty and felt made a fool of by His distractions. His fatherly love only ignited my flames and the anger behind my why intensified. I needed answers like I needed breath, but I found neither. The sky only grew more glorious, almost like a battle of wills. Because I know my limitations between my human capabilities and that of God, I went back inside through the brick walls where death was inevitable and far from pretty. I walked past the breaking souls with my head close to my bleeding heart and the dying baby. That shouldn't even be a sentence. I set my gaze on my breathing baby and turned the music up loud enough to drown out the sounds of hearts breaking down the hall. As the sun moved up through the sky, granting us another day, we moved back up to our home away from home. I hugged every angel like icing filling the naked parts of a cake. My gratitude still knows no bounds. They brought her back. They gave her life again and we are forever indebted. Once she was settled in, my feet carried me to the necessary caffeine I had become dependent on to remain standing.

With new fawn legs, I walked past the room the other family had surrounded just the night before. Again, I lowered my head, respecting the tenderness of the situation. In the elevator, something tugged at me, "Go talk to them." I attempted to shake it off and I focused my gaze on the climbing numbers. But the voice was relentless and eventually I made my way back down to the PICU floor. I was shaking, I was so nervous, but I went in. I greeted the eyes squinting at me. I said that we had seen each other many times, and that I had been praying for them. The baby's mom asked to hug me. I bent down and two stranger moms shared a tearful hug of pain, ache, sorrow and understanding. I explained our life in the hospital and I offered them time, company, cookies and coffee. They declined politely and informed me that their baby had just passed. My heart died again on its 10th life. I was immediately numb all over and like water leaving a faucet, my blood pooled with theirs beneath our embrace. I pulled her mama in tighter, incessantly saying, "I'm sorry." I offered them all I could, knowing damn well it'd never be enough. I exited with my head down, mortified. My timing couldn't have been any worse. Who was that thing who egged me on to go in there? And why in the hell did I listen? In the elevator, I ignited a firestorm and sunk it with my tears.

Back upstairs, I couldn't understand why I was holding my baby while they had just lost theirs. I held my girl tighter, knowing I may not get to forever. If that wasn't a slap in the face that time is of the essence, tomorrow is not promised, I don't know what is. Her breath had become my lifeline, my will to take another breath. Fellow mamas were headed home tonight without their babies. None of this is fair, not even in love and war. My heart still burns for that mama, for every mother who wears these shoes. My message under the door, to the mamas like me, as you sit in this darkness, trying to make sense of the hellish day. When it's finally silent but the chaos is far from over, like that of a broken shower head with no off button. Know this Mama, I know. I don't know you but I'm sitting just feet away from you.

Thinking the same exact thing, feeling the exact same way. Your feelings are validated and no, none of this is okay. I hear your tapping on the wall mama, I'm tapping back. I see you.

CHAPTER 4

$\mathcal{I}$ see you Mama. Your baby has just escaped death by the skin of their teeth that they barely have, yet come morning, you'll be pumping poison into their veins in hopes of keeping them here just a bit longer. I wouldn't wish this hellish life on the devil himself, but here we are Mama. With days that bleed into the night and nights that know no end, forever broken hearted and nowhere near enough coffee, cheers. Weight check and counts were done between four and six in the morning. If she was already awake, I would hit the red button and request to get it all done in hopes that she'd fall back to sleep without interruption. After she'd been poked and prodded, she voiced her anger and it took at least an hour to get her back down. I still attempted to follow that new mom rule - sleep when the baby sleeps, but that rule doesn't apply in the hospital. There were people in and out of the room every 15 minutes, and I felt guilty for sleeping. I felt guilty all of the time. I had this need to be in attendance for every discussion, no matter how minimal. Even if it was just vitals, I needed to know every number. I clung to those numbers for dear life because they were the line for her life. Some of the team let us be if we were sleeping, but other times I woke up to, "Sorry, Mom."

The other day, I had fallen asleep for 10 minutes. I was woken up. After a brief interruption, I slept for another 20 minutes. Again, I was woken up. Mild conversation only made my eyes heavier and I found rest for 15 minutes, but I was woken up. I had finally found a sweet spot on my couch when the cleaning crew came in. At the sound of shaking plastic bags, I threw in the towel. I was at my wits end. She was back on chemo as her team felt there was no immediate reason to break the schedule of treatment, outside of her near-death experience. She was still on TPN but taking sips here and there, more so to wet her whistle and not nearly enough to swallow. Her mucositis was still raging and even yawning would cause her to yelp. She would attempt to open her mouth ever so gently to let out a yawn, expressing her year long exhaustion. The blisters would break open and blood would begin dripping from her mouth. Of all the horrific things to see in this life, watching blood pour from your baby's mouth is something you never come back from. She'd cry out an ache that would break a suit of armor, and yet we were pumping her with more poison. There was no rest for the weary.

She was receiving medications around the clock and after each medication was delivered, it was followed by a flush. There was a tall metal pole with multiple boxes that would blink red and would never stop beeping. My husband, the engineer inside him, couldn't help himself. He had his ways of rigging the room to satisfy our needs as a family, capitalize on as much rest as possible. But after a while, the beeping was enough to make anyone certifiable. Banging my head against the wall and laughing while singing would have made me look completely sane. Timing in the hospital is everything. It is a very well-oiled machine. There were over 20 children on our floor alone, each one of them on a precise medication schedule, and these ladies are sure to keep them all living by following the schedule. Unfortunately, for every family in every room, that meant that our days ran in unison rather than individually. As soon as I would get her down for rest, at least one person, if not five people, would come in. It was a revolving door with team meetings, assessments or medications. There were multiple commercials of mothers putting threatening signs on the front door for delivery people, warding off interruption of her baby sleeping. With the help of some of the nurses, I was able to do something similar in a non-threatening way. But I didn't have much control over the process of keeping her alive or our living situation.

I know my 10 shades of red skin spoke before my mouth would open. No one was at fault. It was simply just the situation that caused difficulty. When young parents are navigating parenthood, everyone says, "Get her on a schedule. It'll help make things easier." There are not many things that can be done to help make hospital living easier, nor is there much of a schedule. There is only "make it through the next few minutes", "hope for tonight", and "pray for a better tomorrow". Unfortunately, that also meant constant interruption. Sleep for all three of us was almost impossible. Privacy was a thing of the past. In our before, if I were using the bathroom, changing clothes or brushing my teeth, she was with me. In the hospital, if I wasn't in the room when someone came in, it felt as if I were unfit as she was in her crib unattended. We were still in the same room. I was just behind a door. I still felt a wave of shame. In our before, it was just the three of us, figuring it all out as best we could. In the hospital, there are over 20 sets of eyeballs on you at one time. It is almost impossible to not feel judged or constantly feel as if your parent card is being red flagged. Like any other new mom, I had barely showered in days and my teeth were desperate for another flavor other than coffee. But no sooner than I ceased an opportunity to take a five second break in the bathroom, with intent to create something resembling a human, than a team of people would enter the room looking for me. It was mortifying to say the least, and more irritating than that of the delivery man who insists on pressing the doorbell despite your many notes to not ring the doorbell. Not to mention, sometimes, it was imperative that I go behind closed doors to lose myself in order to open the door and emerge a human capable of making important decisions. But tickets for mom escapes were few and far between. Therefore, I was beyond sleep deprived, always wreaked of cancer mom, and I was nodding my head as if I had a clue, but truth be told, I barely knew my own name most days.

In the pediatric cancer world, you are constantly working on a team to decide what is best for your child. I'm a difficult person on a good day. I am worthy of love for the most part, but I am not easy to like. Over 1,000 people can attest to that, but I'll be the first. I don't mind working on a team, but when it comes to our child, my husband and I should be the team. When your child has cancer, your team is that of a football organization which is great in terms of saving her life. But the daily different opinions and "answer to" is draining to put it mildly. Because Dakota was on TPN, we would have to log her fluid and food intake. She weighed less than when she had arrived at the hospital back in April. Being on TPN for long periods was hard on the body, so the goal was always to get her to take in nutrition by mouth, to eventually come off of TPN. She needed to hit certain marks for her body to be strong enough to keep fighting. The weaker her body was going into chemo, knowing chemo would completely deplete her, the harder it would be for her body to recover from the crash. But she had developed a fear of anything coming near her mouth. The mucositis, combined with chemo, had caused her to develop a food aversion. She was terrified of pain and awful tastes. Who could blame her? We would attempt to eat all together, hoping to show her the positivity in food. There is no room for a dining room table in a hospital room, so the couch became our family area. With every sip and/or bite she would take in, a party was thrown for encouragement. Nothing about our life or the way we learned to parent was normal. Nothing about our life or the way we parent will ever be normal.

Baths were required nightly to prevent infection. Everything is about preventing infection. Infections lead to fevers. Fevers lead to sepsis. And sepsis leads to death. It was said to me from day one and countless times thereafter, "If cancer doesn't take her, infections could." A bath in the hospital was a series of wet antibacterial cloths used on one part of the body at a time, to be sure not to cross contaminate. She loathed the hospital bath and lost her mind screaming the entire time. I didn't blame her at all. We were wiping her sensitive chemo skin down with lukewarm cloths inside her birdcage. A cold shower would be more appealing. We used a multitude of lotions to help protect her skin from the harsh effects of chemotherapy. We used thick creams to create a barrier between her already damaged skin and the poison that was still oozing out of her. We clothed in her pajamas to keep her as warm as you can be in a hospital, but accessible as even in her sleep she needed to be accessed. Just as we would complete our preparation for yet another sleepless night, there would be a shift change. I have no doubt in my mind that there was a "not it" game played when it came to assigning our room. I don't blame them at all. They had a job and I had a job. Unfortunately, those responsibilities would collide at times. Her medications, vitals, and blood work were all based around time. They had many patients to tend to, but she was my one, my only, my job. She needed rest to heal and to save her strength. But she also needed the 'round the clock interruptions to save her life. It was a balance, like a hefty man riding a unicycle on a tightrope. The lack of sleep and the constant daunting thought that she could die left barely pebbles for patience. Thankfully, our angels in blue, despite not wearing our shoes, chose to walk with us. They carried us through the storms, even when we were the storms. They were awake with us in our insomnia. They never had perfect timing, but they far exceeded patience with their patients.

I should have taken notes because I was losing patience with myself, like wanting to crawl out of my skin over myself. The last few days had been heavy. Like a featherweight carrying the heavyweight up Mount Everest in stilettos heavy. It wasn't Dakota. She was returning to herself by the day. In fact, seeing her smile and hearing her laugh again was what was keeping me afloat. I had cried myself to sleep more times than I could count. My face was lathered in dried, cracking salt. It wasn't one particular thing, but it was everything. Her first Fourth of July was just spent behind brick walls watching the sky sparkle behind glass. We took a wagon ride around the floor where we found an empty room to watch fireworks from a window. We were side-by-side with another inpatient family battling appendicitis. I would have given anything for appendicitis. The wind escaped my sails at the possibility of not being able to go home before we finished this week of chemo and began another. Followed by the chaotic scramble to make it all happen, the process of going "home," even if it was just for a day, maybe two. Topped ever so gently with the discussions of genetic testing. Did we make her like this? Had we done this to her? The words alone caused a tsunami in the back of my throat and made my stomach churn like too thick batter sticking to the sides of the bowl. Sprinkled with the question we avoid like the plague - *another child*? There was no swallowing down that one, only regurgitation. Tie that all in a sailor's knot with insomnia, and a train wreck would resemble Sunday tea in comparison.

I was attempting, with every breath, to make the correct choices for my child who was bravely battling cancer, not sure I had even swallowed that pill yet. There was no thread strong enough to hold me up or keep me together. But there was a possibility we would be going home in the morning. Dakota was healing, bringing tears to every eye who saw her, comparing the sight from just a few days prior. She was eating and drinking, so she was going to be taken off of TPN. She was receiving a Neupogen® shot, which is an injection meant to help her numbers recover. *Home.* That word was still so complicated. Still, with all of its entanglement, it soothed me like a hot cup of cocoa on a cold winter day. Laying with her without restraints, moved me through the moments when she was not breathing. The three of us all in the same bed became my surfboard when we were in the PICU drowning. Home-cooked meals fueled me for the nights when pediatric cancer had me backed into a corner. Breathing in freedom outside of the hospital walls gave me breath in my inability to breathe during discussions about the future of our family. Warm private showers, held me in standing when my knees were buckling. Watching the sunset from a porch rather than a window shined light on each part of our dark shadows. Home was simply *outside of prison walls*. The word reached down into the trenches and pulled me to the surface. I was barely treading water, raging a war on delirium from the overdose of saltwater. But there was a chance we might be going home.

I was sitting on the floor of our room at home, listening to her breathe, another new normal for me. I had become beyond paranoid and scared of everything, everyone. I was terrified she was going to stop breathing or become sick with no way to clear it. I was always on guard for something that would come for her, to take her away. I was petrified all day, every day. I still am. But all day, every day, I would choke down my demons and smile through the suck. I would swing my sword, warding off any darkness that would come within a foot of breathing on her. All the while, despite my natural character to take things quite personally, because I am far too sensitive and overly dramatic. I would not soak in the shots to keep the poison from dripping near her skin. It would come in all forms. Much of it was unintentional. Everyone had an opinion and they were entitled to it, especially since we had been standing on the stage with the lights on. But somewhere along the way of this hell path on earth, I lost the natural right as her mother to know what is best. My opinion meant little in our world of pediatric cancer. I constantly felt belittled as other voices held a higher value. With my forever heart on my sleeve, I carried the shame for going against the grain. I chose to not smile pretty and nod in agreement, making me all the more difficult and a burden. I could see it in their eyes, despite the silent treatment. They had become beyond agitated at their scrutiny due to my resistance. We all had our toes dug in and we were pushing against the brick wall on opposite sides. I am fire on my best day, but I am put out quickly as I associate more with a wet mop. I wanted to cry, scream, die in the fetal position, and run all at the same time. But I stood my ground, a lone soldier on the battlefield. This was much bigger than me and I was determined to make certain this didn't become about them. My eyes were stern, but I politely smiled. My skin told a much different story as I couldn't hide its cherry red color, unveiling my truth despite my every effort.

I held it together, until I couldn't. Sometimes those four walls just engulfed me. My wings had been clipped. She was bound and he was tied up in the corner, the three of us prisoners to our life. Thousands of spiders danced on my skin, teasing me with their tickling feet that felt more like tiny knife stabs. I had to get us out. There must be a window with bars we could slide through. The restriction was suffocating. Our wings were breaking through the flesh of our shoulder blades. Maybe through the vent, we could crawl like mice through the tunnel. We couldn't breathe, as if plastic bags covered our heads. This is the path most taken with the best chance at survival. This was the best chance at life outside of this life, but this wasn't living. It was a slow death in our every attempt not to die. Our arms knew no rest from swinging our swords. We were always in the fight, defending. With every breath, we were attempting to keep the three of us alive. All day and every day with no reprieve. We fought sleep because we didn't know how to lay down our swords. I refused to close my eyes. Death would surely come for us if I let it down just an inch. But we were already dying, a slow death, attempting to survive. Listening to her breathe was my way of swinging. I had to keep swinging. With every scream she belted, because poison was burning her from the inside out. I held onto this, on the floor watching her breathe. Each time she was snapped back from looking out the window by her tubes and wires, I held on to this. Every episode of projectile vomiting followed by her head buried in my shoulder, I clung to this. Each bath of tears we soaked one another in out of sheer pain and agony, I held on to this. I held onto these daydreams, like three greasy fingertips on the edge of a cliff in a thunderstorm. I held on, telling myself, if we can just get through this. If we could just get through this, we could swing on the swing. We could take a ride in the wagon outside, allowing the earth to kiss our wounds. Maybe we could pretend to forget, even if only for a few seconds.

I once dreamed big. I literally planned years ahead of time. My dreams were made small. My dreams became everyday things that we all take for granted. A morning stroll with a takeout cup of coffee. Falling in love with the way the sun shines glitter on my baby's skin. The freedom of having the ability to go outside. Being snuggled up under a blanket, kept warm by love. Cooking with a glass of wine in one hand and spatula in the other. Mr. Sinatra serenading me, whispering all of the things the woman inside me needs to hear. Sleeping in a bed with the three of us all together, intertwined and never close enough. I stopped longing for plane rides or postcard views. I crave only the simple things, the little things that have always been the big things. Before cancer, her feet touched the floor without worry. She played in the dirt and I held no fear. She was exposed to germs without a gasp. Until everything became a threat to her life. Nothing was safe and all things, including air, became dangerous. I didn't know what tomorrow would bring, let alone the next five minutes. All I knew was the present, our current moment. I'd never again take this life for granted. I learned to be grateful for every moment despite selfishly wanting more than just a moment. I knew we may only have this moment and I held on.

We headed into clinic to assess her recovery and ability to keep pushing forward, holding on. Despite the win that her numbers were on the climb, I was feeling lost. I felt I was wading in 12 feet of water. I'm under five feet tall and there were rocks in my boots. My baby, who had only been in this world for a few months, was fighting for her life. Isn't that an oxymoron? She had and would continue to endure a pain meant to break grown men. Her hair continued to snap, making frail twigs look like 100-year-old oak trunks. Her skin was so pale it made white sheets look ivory. Her natural born fierceness was taunting her to run full force, but she was held captive in every way. We both watched another infant in pure cafeteria jealousy. She was Dakota's age, not tied to a pole, free as a bird. She was touching the floor and as my cancer mom chest tightened in fear of germs, I realized that her behavior was completely normal in their normal. My heart broke for both of us, as it was a visual reminder of our clipped wings. The number three had been everywhere for weeks. It was like a blinking light, fighting to always be in my line of vision. I had been avoiding it, terrified of its significance. It was relentless and only shined brighter at my shunning. Its persistence kept we me awake in my already awake. I began asking it, "Three more months, three years old? What are you trying to tell me?" Was that all the time she had left? I picked a fight with God.

I was instructed early on to stay off of the internet, but I couldn't help myself. Angel number three means *we are here, we hear you*. It is the angels saying *we are working on it. Stay the path. Keep pushing forward. We are protecting you*. I saw their faces, our angels in the sky, and I cried happy tears. I rolled my chest towards Dakota's head and a peace washed over me like a wave. My faith has always been a work in progress. I am forever far too far from grace. Our turn in this life made me angry in a way I struggled to shake. It left me broken with no chance at repairs. Her fight had gifted me with a fight I'll never win, but I will spend my life fighting. Despite my fury, I leaned in and as always, He held me up. His light shined through her and reminded me that I was never truly alone. Like vomit climbing the ladder in my esophagus, I felt compelled to speak, and to speak loudly. He created me to physically embody the size of a child yet to hold a megaphone deep inside with no volume down button. He has a quirky sense of humor, that Man in the sky. I cannot tell you, the many times I had heard, "I don't believe in God but tonight I spoke to Him. I had been told, "I don't pray but tonight I prayed." With a full heart, I grabbed my chest, closed my eyes and embraced His hug all around me. The night kidnapped me in a black trash bag. My toes scraped the bottom of the ocean floor, but their wings held me up. Despite the devil in her veins, our angels were with us. I couldn't see them, but I could feel them. I whispered into the dark of the night, asking them to not let us go, for in them, we were not lost but found.

Even in the lost and found, the box itself could get chaotic. Cancer holds a multitude of characteristics. Lying is his main character flaw. Just as quickly as she was laughing, dancing and shining bright, she was down and out. Her pink shade turned gray and the vomiting replaced her giggle. Her ballerina legs grew tired and she only wanted to lay down. That is the deceit of cancer. As the light starts to warm your soul to at least room temperature, he creeps in and turns a summer day into mid-February. As if the whiplash from almost "normal" to warrior paint on wasn't enough, she began screaming a scream that only meant one thing. Her head was hot on my chest like a cigarette burn. She was twisting her torso like a worm, writhing as if to physically explain the turmoil inside. She began pulling away from me with eyes closed and I begged her to keep breathing. Lips, please don't turn blue. Her temperature read 99, teasing me like the calm before the storm. I laid her down next to me in bed and selfishly found breath within her breath on my neck. I scanned every inch of her, searching for a sign, something to tell me to make a move. She was barely awake and her bobble head was begging me to just go start the car. I was stealthy taking her temperature, being sure not to wake her, but craving its numbers like a frantic feen. She was on the cusp, but not over yet. I watched her chest rise and fall and gaged her skin, pleading with her to tell me what she needed me to do. If I went to the ER, I would risk exposing her to germs that could kill her. If I waited too long, I could be just a second too late and lose her. When she woke up, she let out a shrill I knew all too well. It was a raspy, chain smoker cry like after she had been intubated. Her throat sounded like rubbing sand paper between fingertips. Mucositis maybe? But she was drinking, swallowing and she wasn't struggling to breathe. Her legs grazed my stomach and I felt her chill, so I wrapped just her lower half in a blanket. I kissed her cheek and felt the flame burning beneath the surface. I placed my hand on her chest. She was still breathing. She began letting out a soft cry as if she were holding back. She doesn't soft cry. She was up every hour on the hour and I knew something was definitely wrong. The ER was germ-infested and therefore life-threatening. It was 5:00 in the morning and clinic didn't open until 8:00. If we could just hold on until then. The universe must have heard me as no sooner than those thoughts ran across my mind did her body spike. I packed a bag, frantically attempting to buy us time, not knowing how much time we had. We were above the fever line, but it was only 6:30. I pushed through that last hour and a half, anxiously waiting for the clock to strike 8:00. I was wrong and I knew I was wrong, but no decision in the situation was right. I gave myself an internal beating for waiting. With my head pounding and my eyes almost swollen shut, I got us in the car and on the way to the hospital, praying she'd be okay.

She was far from okay, battling a fever and her numbers were low, which meant she could not fight off anything. We were immediately admitted and before I could blink, she was hooked up to a pole with multiple medications running through her. She wouldn't eat or drink, but she was able to find sleep. It felt like déjà vu, and we were on the precipice of spiraling once again. I knew she wasn't okay and I waited. Had I waited too long? She was not okay, but she was exactly where she needed to be. While she found rest and fought to fight the battle that was taking place inside her, I cooked up a storm inside myself. She was rolling at three weeks, standing at two months and she would be 10 months this upcoming week. She wanted to walk, but she had been tied to a pole more often than not these last few months, crucial developmental months. She would attempt to move, but the tubes would pull her back like a bungee cord. I would make myself beyond annoying to her team in order to give her as much slack as possible, slack on the leash attached to my baby. Sick. She would feel it pull and shoot me this look, begging me for freedom like a dog on a chain. Some days, she just wasn't up to it because she didn't feel good and had little to no strength. Cancer was holding her back and the drugs she was on, meant to save her life, have long term effects. The effects are not guaranteed, but forewarned. The gift that keeps on giving. The list was endless - memory loss, inability to focus, infertility, heart defects, inhibited growth, just to name a few. We were attempting to kill poison with poison and this was protocol. We were in a fight with no end. If she makes it to school someday, she could find frustration trying to remember, despite her natural intelligence. One day, we could be in a dressing room and she may be staring at her reflection in the mirror, disgusted by her scars despite her undeniable beauty. She may never know the joy of being a mommy, discovering the very reason for her breath here on this earth.

While the breath was still in her lungs, I made it my mission to stay in front of the storms ahead. I would give her brain every chance to blossom beautifully. I would be sure her every muscle had the strength it needed to thrive. I was bound and determined that if we were ever gifted that moment in the dressing room, she would know that she was the most breathtaking angel the good Lord has ever sent down here. She would know no shame of her warrior scars or the life she has been given. It would be a life of damage over death, but she would be here. My only wish, but at what cost? Being her mama is the greatest gift of my life. The question of another had come up far too many times for my own discomfort level. Before cancer, we had every intention of having another baby, a little brood. Everything had changed, including who we were as people and our desires. I would never do to another child what we have had to do to Dakota. I know that statement alone makes many want to reach through the page and scream at me or worse. I may not have been the root cause and we may never know the why. But watching her fight to live hasn't been fair to her or to anyone. If I can prevent another soul from enduring this hell, I will. Our life had become a story, a journey of grief in all forms. I would still smile, dance and receive the best hugs, hugs that could heal the devil's wrath. I threw glitter at the wall all day, in places that know no light.

Sometimes creating shiny meant dancing around the room like a fool. Other times it meant holding her for hours on end, leaving us both soaked in sweat. When she slept, I allowed myself to be human. I physically felt all of the things and said all of the things I'd been choking down. When I was with her, I was sure to smile through my tears. I didn't let her know that in my head I was reminding myself to savor the moment. There was something inside me always reiterating that I may never know the passing moment again. Inside, I was a broken that could not be fixed, but all she knew was my smile. Cancer and chemo were both chipping away at her, bit by bit. Cancer and chemo were both bleeding out of me, two slices at a time. The clock was ticking all too fast. Our future was a blur, like fog in the mountains the morning after a rain storm. We were constantly tucking and rolling, army crawling under lit barbed wire. We had wet noodles for legs, yet we were hoping to stand and face tomorrow. There was a time we were too sure of tomorrow. We had the next 10 years and beyond planned out and nothing would hinder our map out on paper as neither one of us knew how to fail. I prided myself on being all three - a mother, a wife and a career woman. I never imagined caregiver would be a part of my resume. In our before, I strived every single day to give all three roles the best version of me, wore myself thin. I knew I would inevitably fail and fall short, but I'd die trying anyway. There were never enough hours or enough arms. I was too content in my life. I never felt more like myself than when I became Dakota's mama. I loved being a wife to my husband, building together from the ground up. I was one of those people who could honestly say that I loved my job, even on the hard days. I believed in my work, despite getting home late sometimes. I hated when her eyes were closed when I walked through the door. Sometimes so close to the endzone, but fell flat on my face at the five-yard line.

I was always letting someone down. If I didn't stick to the timeline exactly, I would drop the ball somewhere. I always felt like I was letting my husband down. He never spoke the words but his gaze on me had changed. I longed to give him all of me, but I was in a tug of war with myself to give myself to every space needed with drops to spare. Not being all that I needed to be to everyone chewed me up inside. This is a woman's turmoil, the demons that eat her alive. I thought I was exhausted then, but I was happy. When cancer plowed through our door, I never went back to being that woman. It wasn't even an option. The night of diagnosis, I told my husband that I would never leave her and he said that he already knew. I had spent every single day since April 24th with my daughter and I have never regretted one second. It was excruciating. She had *boo boos* I couldn't heal. Our situation was all-consuming, an endless tornado with no exit sign. But I was with her every second of every single day. There was not a moment that I had missed. I watched her eyes open with the sunrise and I watched them close with the darkness of the night. She knew that I was always there and she would never know anything else. I loathed our life. My own death would be floating on marshmallows in the sky, sipping on sprinkles in comparison. But there was nowhere else I could ever be. I was still wearing myself too thin, tissue paper under the weight a rolling pin. There were still not enough seconds in the day, yet the days were everlasting. I was not the octopus I needed to be, but more so a giraffe on a pool float in the middle of the ocean. She had my every, just a few inches short, efforts. We were on borrowed time all of the time. I would watch the clock like a sprinter's gaze challenges the stopwatch. I'd hang my head in shame for every minute prior to this life that I had selfishly taken for granted. I had it all, and like a greedy gremlin, I wanted more. I had nothing to complain about, yet griped like a wealthy man at a white cloth restaurant crushing peanuts on the floor. With kettle chips on my shoulders, I had something to prove - I could do it all. But I now had nothing and someone to save, a job I was almost guaranteed to fail miserably. But I would kill myself trying. My job title now read, "Dakota's mom". My job description was, "don't let her die".

She was my number one priority. No one and nothing came before her. I had made people irate. There were countless eyerolls, scoffs, certain fingers and the colorful words that come with it. People that were once sewn into our picture became a black dot somewhere off in the distance. There was shredded threading in the space between. I didn't blame them. I didn't expect anyone to understand. Without wearing shoes as I do, there is no comprehension, and there is absolutely no comparison. I have owed over one million apologies, yet I didn't have two pennies to rub together. I didn't have the time to spare, as every second was being spent on her. My patience was long gone, like a spec of glitter drifting out to sea. My empathy was that of a nun teaching Catholic school during a blizzard with a trigger-happy ruler. I had more words to spew than that of every version of the Bible and yet I grew mute. I craved touch more than I longed for wine and chocolate, but the thought of breath near me made me carsick. I was in such a constant state of anger, that a paperclip that kissed the floor was like a landslide and I was operating a tricycle going downhill. There was no sanity in our insanity. We were barricaded by four walls, hanging on the words, "She could die." If sanity was still being served, I would check for a pulse. We had died but we were still living, making failed attempts at keeping her alive. We were busy saving her life and the only message I could get out was, *leave your message at the beep*. After a blood and platelet transfusion, she perked up with a smile that stole the sun's shine. Seconds after our shoulders left our ears, we were told she was well enough to begin more chemo. It was defeating in that less than 24 hours ago, we were facing down possible life-threatening infections. She was down and out and no sooner than her finding her footing again, we were going to bring her right back down. It was a rollercoaster ride that made whiplash move at a snail's pace. The highs and lows were emotionally exhausting and there was no time to process, as the only mode was go. It was time, time to put on our war paint. The stadium walls trembled at the base of her theme song from *Moana*, "How Far I'll Go." She was a champion with her satin hood up. Her head down, eyes up, fists high and quick feet. She took in deep breaths, tasting the salt dripping from her brow. Her entrance music blaring *Hillsong's* "Oceans." The crowd's screams were drowning out her thoughts. Cancer was pacing in the corner. I love the part where she would unrobe. It is a pivotal moment, the breath before the cowboy pulls his gun in a draw. They would pat her down while her gaze was set on the center of the room up ahead. Her coach's voice was putting a bug in her ear. Her hand was on the rope. This was it. She ducked down low, entering the ring. There was only one way in and one way out. Her face was painted with grit. My fighter, only 10 months old, weighing in at 12 pounds. Adorned in a Minnie dress with her head on a swivel. Her daddy taught her that. Her blue eyes that could kill. Take that, Satan. Her legs were like spaghetti, but she could out race a cheetah. Her breath was the sound that silenced the dome. She stripped down to her diaper, baring her every earned warrior scar. Her eyes squinted down at her devices embedded under her skin, but she kept her chin up. I bugged her ear with, "Keep breathing, I'm right here. You got this!" The bell rang, ding, ding, ding. Her fists opened as if to throw the first punch, but she caressed his face. She held his face in her palm. She was fighting with love.

CHAPTER 5

She had a lumbar puncture, which is where chemotherapy is injected directly into the spine in hopes of preventing cancer cells from infiltrating the spinal fluid and blood/brain barrier. Her procedure went well and her temperament hadn't changed. She was eating and drinking without hesitation, still giving the sun a run for her money. The seas were calm and the next storm was funneling up ahead. We were able to go home in the interim to capitalize on the strength and build up momentum. I was remembering the moment after the doctors placed her on my chest. I asked if I could feed her immediately. I pulled her into me and she latched, fed. I had filled a deep freezer with milk in no time at all. Around her five-month mark, I began making all of her food. I purchased fruits and vegetables directly from the farm. I was blending and filling mason jars like it was my job. She loved the awakening of her tastebuds. I was floating on a donut float in a private pool with an umbrella drink, lost in my daydream. Then, the winds picked up and the under tow swept me out into the hurricane. Like a dark wave, I was remembering sitting on the red couch of the red room on the fifth floor of our treating hospital. We were barely minutes into our new life, discussing the layout of the next two years of this life ahead. One of the doctors unintentionally crushed my soul by stating that my blender and cloth diaper days were dead and over. I didn't know then just how dead. It wasn't long before our impressive feeding streak would come to a screeching halt. Chemotherapy had annihilated the bumps on her tongue that had provided the pleasures of food. It also gifted her with an upset stomach and an incessant taste of vomit in the back of her throat. Clusters of blisters like heads on cauliflower grew like wildflowers throughout her digestive tract. They would gush open and permit only the taste of pus and blood to whet her palate. With food and drink off the table, her weight would drop dramatically.

Skin and bones don't stand a chance in going toe to toe with cancer. TPN, her intravenous nutrition, became the only item on the menu. Days turned to weeks, and weeks flowed into a month. The longer she was on TPN the more potential for damage it held. I was dancing, singing and pleading from my knees for her to take in just a few sips of PediaSure®. I recorded ounces in on a whiteboard, like a gold star on the chalkboard. Those ounces held the same swaying power of the numbers documented after blood was drawn. They were the granted wish of a few days home or the added days to our grounding in the hospital. My life raft came in the form of her sitting in her highchair in the kitchen of my parents' home. There was a Gerber teething cookie, like thin cardboard, laying solo on the tray. She picked it up in her tiny hand and brought the tasteless box cutout to her lips. She opened her broken mouth and bit down. I immediately began balling hysterically and jumping up and down as if she had just scored the final goal with seconds left in the game because to me, she just did. After feeding just seconds into life, to becoming petrified of food and drink. This was a small win that was a big win, increasing strength and generating momentum. They were right in that we needed the space outside of those hospital walls to regain some physical and emotional power. The in-between was always over faster than the snap of two fingers. The feeding party was over before we could throw our hands into the air, as it was time to go back in and suit up.

With the bags under our eyes showcasing our lack of sleep and our bodies using our shackles as armor, we were as ready as we could be. Her body wasn't ready yet. She hadn't had enough sleep or enough food, and her numbers were too low to begin swinging again. Steroids, the necessary evil. The sword that holds the power to take it away but doesn't hold enough power to keep it all away. The evil who summons other demons to take over the body and wreak havoc. The dark creature who paints her face a terrifying shade of red, holds captive her sleep and turns her belly inside out. One would think that the mind adjusts to the chaos and the blows eventually don't cave the house in, but every hit was detrimental. The mental game in this war was taking years off our life with little effort. Each time she didn't make counts, a previous wound reopened and a new one was born. There was a constant game of tug of war being played in our heads. It was imperative to remain on schedule with little hiccups to hold on to the light at the end of the tunnel. But being in the hospital had begun to feel safer than being in our in-between, as being bound to the pole meant we were still in the fight. My head was buried in my chest with my hood up as it was the only physical hole I could crawl into. I didn't want to look at anyone, let alone use my voice to speak out of fear that the venom I would unintentionally spew would harm a helpless victim. I had to pull myself inside myself in order to taste the reality of our reality. I was careful not to swallow down the poison, but with the chemicals fuming on my tongue, I had to be alone to keep everyone else safe. It was a poor excuse for a defense mechanism and a failed attempt at survival mode. But this was my way of staying alive, hoping to keep her alive. Evil preys on the weak and I was barely able to lift my chin off of the floor. Chief was our first baby before our baby came. His world had been flipped upside down as much as ours had. This was no fairer to him than it was to us. He deserved better than this turmoil and we had made the decision to give him better than us. The darkness thickened with our decision and it was becoming more difficult to see through the multiple losses, let alone breathe through the grief. After multiple nights consumed with mourning, but no rise of the morning, comparable to years 14 through 18 of an emo teenager, it was time to try again.

With anchors tied to our ankles, we were trying to find the surface in a pool filled with angst and all of the demons. It was a cesspool filled with snakes, crocodiles, sharks, tarantulas and zombies. We were in our birthday suits caked in vulnerability. Hold your nose and jump in. If I wasn't pacing, I was packing. We were like businessmen living out of suitcases, without the snazzy clothes on wheels. Our beat-up duffle bags were stained with coffee and chemo. Our hotel made a shredded tent in a dark alleyway look like a five-star resort. Would we stay or would we go? I was consumed with dread. There were not enough paper bags to restore my breath. I was overwhelmed with an untouchable ache in my heart, like witnessing children's bodies line the concrete after an unexpected storm. A wave of grief was drowning me, living briefly in one world while preparing for the worst in the other. The waiting was a padded room in and of itself. The seconds like hours, minutes like days, and hours like weeks. There were no nails left to chew off or strands of hair to pull out. The top numbers came in and it was a maybe. A rack of basketballs were rubbing my esophagus raw. My heart was a broken drum hammering the floor. Across the room, the nurses' arms flew up in the air. Touchdown. Her numbers were good and we were being admitted, to beat her down. I swallowed down relief and fear like a shot of tequila without the chaser. His laugh was ringing in my ear causing my neck to twitch. I was having flashbacks of blood pouring from her mouth and her lips turning blue. I could hear her choking on chemo and gasping for breath. There was a crystal ball floating within an arm's reach. Its insides were swirling like the inside of a tornado. The blurred images were giving me a headache and making it hard to stand. Just before I could see a clear picture, it shattered on the floor in pieces. If this was a premonition, we were clearly headed for disaster.

It was an out of body experience watching us make our way upstairs. Our home away from home and our battlefield with no mini bar. My stomach was in knots, twisting like a wrung-out rag. My head was in a drunk daze and it hadn't stopped spinning. It was time to return to my body and face the fight. There was no choice. We had to jump in, sink or swim. We stood no chance. We were almost immediately sinking. She screamed and hit my chest because I couldn't feed her. She was banging on me because I am the one who is supposed to make it better. I constantly felt like the worst mother ever. I could not begin to fathom her confusion. I'd be laying into me too if I were her. I was throwing a party when she brought a cardboard cookie to her mouth one day, then denying her food the next. The guilt made a knife to the stomach seem like a massage. Across the hall, she perked up because she was never in the hall and shiny things were captivating. If she only knew that these things were dull and there were true shiny things she hadn't even seen yet.

The ladies in blue were lining the perimeter of the morgue-esque table. Time would stop in this room and the temperature made an igloo look like a sauna. I held her close with my lips to her ear. I told her that I loved her, demanded that she keep breathing and begged her come back to me. I laid her down feeling as if I were placing her inside a coffin. I was fighting the urge of my arms to pull back, forcing myself to let go. With tear-filled eyes, I told the room to take care of my girl. They assured me that they would, and I believed them, despite choking on the memory of the last time.

I shut the door behind me and with my belly button touching my back, I silently made deals with God. I curled my face into her blanket, intoxicating myself with the smell of her, my only home. Without her in my arms, I felt as if I had lost a limb. Waiting in the empty space was suffocating and the elevator walls were closing in. Internally, I was scaling the walls during the fall, losing sight of up and down. My nails stopped clawing at the concrete when I heard her cry. The songbird to my ears, I couldn't help but smile ear to ear. My feet pounded into the ground but never quick enough. After a lifetime apart, my limb was sown, eliminating the seams. She threw her body back like the arch of a body enduring the lash of a whip. It presented like agony in its most grotesque form. Her face was that shade of red that only comes from hours slathered in baby oil, on broil under the sun. Another lashing came on harder than the one before and her head severed from my chest. Her shoulder blades became engulfed in a passionate kiss, like her flesh was being torn from the bone. It was an ungodly sight despite the whispers around me echoing the word normal. If this was normal, what was the latter? She was swollen, resembling a tiny Buddha. Her eyes were barely open as if the daylight was blinding. I was screaming for answers in the chaotic noise of the word *normal* being tossed around like confetti. My broken warrior was searching for my gaze through sliced eyes. With her hand on my chest, she told me, "I'm still breathing Mama."

I knew it would only get worse before it would get better, and then it would get worse again. I was grateful in that I knew just her taking breath in my arms in that moment was a gift. Still, I desperately needed to make it better despite knowing all too well that I couldn't make it better. I was climbing the walls, making every attempt to fail her in the least way possible. She finally found some rest after scaling me like a baby cub with wolves howling down below. When she woke up, she was slightly less swollen and I could see her baby blues I had been missing. When I would wake up in the morning, the first thing I wanted to see, was her face. Her big blues, like mother ocean, call me home. They find me almost immediately and it's love at first glance every single time. Her priceless smile would melt the ice I had become. My heart leaped on a trampoline at the sight of her beauty. She summoned me to come close by curling her pointer finger up. Her hand kissed my cheek and there was nowhere else I'd rather be. I leaned into her as she leaned into me. I rubbed my face against hers, with hers against mine. We both would coo and smile, a joy dreams are made of. We snuggled, wrapped in our fuzzy blankets, intertwined within one another. I held her close in her spot on my left shoulder, as we became one. Love you more. We hummed to one another, speaking our own love language.

The other day in clinic, a nurse said as I walked by, "It's so weird to see you without her on you. She's always attached to you." I smiled and immediately missed her already. She was a piece of me. Another nurse was watching her and me just being us in our room. She said, "You guys are really close, aren't you?" I didn't know what to say at first because I didn't know anything else. We were close, and for us, I don't know that there's any other way. She grew inside me and fed from me. Just months later, we were told she may not be here long. We have clung to one another desperately, cherishing every second. We had been facing down death together hoping to live side by side. We have lived within one another's breath. She is my best friend, my favorite person and my hero. She is everything we all should be. She is my home and my whole world. To be close to her is never close enough. My love for her knows no bounds. Not even death could keep us apart. I am hers and she is mine. Her 24-hour chemo had begun. The scary part was not watching the neon yellow poison pump into her. The fear that stole my breath was the storm it was brewing while flowing through her veins to potentially take her breath. No sooner than the yellow kiss of death stopped flowing, did the effects of its love present themselves. Despite fluids being pumped into her like a waterfall, she began with some redness downstairs and drooling. With cotton balls in her diaper to gage the clearing of the poison from her body, the upcoming crash was inevitable.

The crash was a site not meant to be seen by human eyes, but here we were, witnessing the devil's purposeful accident on our child. Her baby soft skin was ripped open, exposing her flesh meant for the inside. She was lathered in blisters, leaving her "down there" and chest completely raw. The scene was riveting and paralyzing to put it politely. Not only was she smiling through excruciating pain, but her wide-open skin threatened her life due to risk of infection. We were attempting to put out fires in every inch of our box, all while being sure not to be consumed by the blaze ourselves. Meanwhile, her supporters attended a fundraiser in her honor. A dear friend of mine who has loved me through all of my colorful phases, is a tattoo artist. She held a day at her shop to honor Dakota's fight. People near and far gathered to permanently express their love for Dakota and their admiration for her strength. There is something incredibly intoxicating and healing about the slight pain of a needle pulsing into your flesh. It is a release of the inside depths finding the surface. A wave of peace overpowers the buzzing and permits a ride through a water barrel, showering with clarity. After a few hours, the numbness becomes exactly what was needed without the knowing that it was in fact needed. The piece of art memorializing significance becomes a pivotal experience in itself. At the end, the skin showcases the darkness on the inside that when brought to light is beauty in its truest form. Dakota was enduring a darkness birthed in a place made up of only death. People were giving her darkness light, thereby creating beauty. We were on fire, but the world was seeing our light.

Through her dark, she found her light and spoke it to me. She couldn't use words, but she was sure her voice was heard. She had stopped drinking despite my failed attempts at bottle offers throughout the day. She responded with a blatant "no". She told me in the only way she could, "no Mama, it hurts". Heard. She wanted to snuggle more than play. She'd tuck a blanket that we called her "woob" into her hands, insert her thumb, and fall into me. Like hot cocoa on my skin, I selfishly held onto the moment, a moment too long. I watched the change play out. Like a pit, I was slowly being hollowed out as she was falling down the hole while shards of glass sliced through her. It was like watching a tractor trailer slide on black ice into the 10 cars up ahead. An inevitable collision, and there was not a damn thing I could do to stop it. I knew the worst was yet to come. Like sitting in the seat beside the person impaled and sandwiched, stuck between life and death. There was nothing I could do, but I had to do this to her to have a chance at keeping her here, alive. I loathed and appreciated the fight all the same. It was killing me to watch her battle, but I was grateful for the chance to give her life. The silence of the chaos was deadly, but her screams gave me hope as it meant that she was still here.

Through her screams, I made every attempt at getting her to take something in. It was my desperate attempt to keep her from relying on IV nutrition. But she made it very plain that she would not take anything by mouth. She did everything outside of taking my teeth from my mouth to be sure she was heard. With each refusal, another piece of me broke. Like a branch full of cracks and a caterpillar takes a stroll, it didn't take much, but it was more than enough. Her body was a brutal shade of red, raw and blanketed in burns. She was engulfed in flames with her skin peeling back layer by layer. She was torn open, seeping and she smelled of burnt flesh. The chemicals leaking through her pores singed the hairs in our noses. The toxins were melting her, slowly transitioning her flesh into liquid. I cried with her every time I had to wipe "down there". I felt as if I were bathing her in acid. Immediately after scorching her, I slathered her in the concrete, a cream regimen to create a barrier. It was a shot in the dark to decrease the amount of chemicals kissing her baby skin. She cried out at my gloved touch and my soul took one of its last breaths. I was alone more than I wasn't, which opened space for swimming in my head. I scanned through my phone and realized the essence of my alone. I had been hearing daily, "I'm here if you need anything." But there were too many to count, that I hadn't heard from. I told myself it was because they didn't know what to say. But the real truth was, I didn't know what to say. They were busy continuing on with their lives as they were still on play. Our lives had stopped. We were on pause. They couldn't look because it was too much, but we weren't given a choice. We had become redundant, the same song on a different day. What I wouldn't give to be so blissfully naïve. They had placed a piece of silver duct tape on my forehead. With a black Sharpie, they had written the word "drama." Was this dramatic enough for you? I wouldn't wish this life on anyone. Even in the love and hate, no eyes should see this or hear this side of hell. It was better that they stay away and that I distanced us. There was no need to disturb anyone with our drama. She was still here and that is all that truly mattered. We were alone in our never-ending night, but we still held light.

She was being swallowed whole by the darkness. She couldn't help but be all over the place, like a ball inside a pin ball machine. One minute she was smiling and laughing. The next, she was on a path of destruction and she couldn't settle herself.

She was terrified of anything that came within a five-mile radius of her mouth. She had hit her wall, full speed ahead with no helmet on. She was trying desperately to find ground. She would hum, grind her teeth and make failed attempts at deep breaths. Even her lollipop thumb wasn't doing the trick as it was dipped in acid too. Her body was writhing like a boa constrictor and her screams mimicked the act of her being ripped apart inside. I pulled the trigger in an attempt to end the misery. Pain medication filled me with fear and guilt. It made a pit form in my stomach the size of the Grand Canyon. But within minutes, she was herself. She wanted to stand and look out of the window. She attempted to walk, jump, eat and even drink. I was taken aback by the night and day, still tormented by the tug of war game with myself. Only on pain medications was she able to function. It became a permanent punch I took to the throat that never healed. Drifting back to reality, away from my daydream nightmare and into my actual nightmare, I had noticed that her dressing was opening. Immediately, alarms were sounding, lights were blinking and red flags were popping up everywhere. Another risk of infection as if her open flesh wasn't enough. Talk about a kick when down. Her dressing had to be sealed as it exposed the hole in her chest which was a direct line to her blood stream. It took three of us to hold her down. She kicked, screamed and yelled out in protest. Everyone was sweating, getting a weeks' worth of cardio in these few minutes. She couldn't stop screaming, until I picked her up. That sniffle was her way of saying *I'm still trying to get myself together; give me a few more minutes*. I held her close and rocked her. Within minutes, she was asleep. I couldn't help but stare at her deep in peace. I grazed my fingertips gently over skin like cotton. I was thinking, *He wouldn't bring her here, do all of this, just to take her away, right?* She was moving mountains with deep valleys on deck. I stared out of the window, watching the world go by, begging the sky to please let her stay.

Despite my cries and her clear physical break down, we were moving forward with another dose of 24-hour chemo. These are the necessary choices we had to make that took pieces of our soul that will never breathe life again. She had a fuzzy stuck to her lip, so I tried to pull it off. She pulled away from me and began to wail. I scooped her up and told her it was okay, but it wasn't. The fuzzy wasn't stuck to her lip, it was stuck to a blister on her lip. With my will to live tied to a rope in knots buried in what was left of my stomach. The word mucositis curled between my feet and pulled my life away from my body hand over hand. My heart was a sunken ship, dredging up the ocean floor. Another lump formed in my throat, this one the size of a beach ball filled with rocks. I laid her down to get a better look, only to find two more blisters. I bit down hard to keep the dam from breaking and immediately informed her team. I was secretly hoping this would delay treatment by a few days to give her time to heal. But my red balloon on a string was popped with one prick. We had to keep going, onward and downward. Tomorrow morning, she would be injected with poison for 24 hours. A catheter would be placed inside her, and with my hand gripping my ribs, I was desperately hoping we would dodge another horrendous night of pushing.

I could still hear her screams as they pushed over and over again that night, a living nightmare I will never forget. The hairs on my neck, like an army of soldiers, stood at attention. In the days to come, she would stop drinking and eating completely. The blisters would coat her mouth and lips, resembling bloody cottage cheese. That was only a visual of what we would be able to see. The inside of her would blind eyes at the sight. No child should endure this and no parent should witness this. Pain medications used casually in the streets would permit my baby sleep. She would wake often with the inability to swallow, choking on her own secretions. Drool would pour like a waterfall cascading down her chin, better out than in. Blood-like tar would paint her lips like red lipstick. Her lips would stick together while she slept and would rip apart as she woke. She would be inconsolable as the meds wore off and she'd stare at me blankly as the meds kicked in. I know more than I should because we were just here less than a few weeks ago. I've been dreading facing days like this since. We were all about to travel waters we've already damn near drowned in. We were on a kayak in a tsunami, with kindling for paddles. We were prepared with blankets as life jackets, foreseeing the capsize. Like sailing on a sunny and 75-degree day, in the Virgin Islands, drink in hand. But headed straight for the eye of the storm ahead. White foam lathering the waves, calling our names. This is the very place we almost lost her. Where I held her in my arms, living out my worst fear. This is where she lost breath for the second time, but I was almost certain, it was the last time. We couldn't near that line again. Like a riptide, the evil twin sister of the ocean was sucking me in. I dug my heels into the wet stand, searching for driftwood. But her rope lassoed my ankles as her mean girl laugh bellowed in my ear. I positioned myself in a deep squat, planting firm on land. She whispered, "Come play."

There was a game we had to play that none of us wanted to play. I held her down as they repositioned her catheter, begging God for the most minimal number of pushes. With gym socks in my throat, I kept my gaze on her. She looked back at me with a look that drowned me in guilt. The guilt was like a plastic bag over my head filled with salt water. I deserved every swallow. Her big water-filled blues looked up at me, begging me to make it stop. I told her over and over again that it was going to be okay. But I was lying through gritted teeth. I sang the *ABC's*, shooshing my way through her bellows. I told her I was right here, not that my being there made any of it better. I told her I was so proud of her and commended her bravery. All while a plastic tube was being shoved in a place where plastic tubes should never be shoved. The way she was looking at me let me know that I was letting her down. No matter if I went up or down, left or right. If I made circles or figure eights, I was failing her miserably at every turn. After the episode came to an end, I held her, attempting to make it better. I bounced, rocked and rubbed my face all over hers. I kissed every inch of space that didn't expose open flesh. She made me earn her lips as I had just assisted in her pain. I hate me too, Boo. Eventually, she threw in the towel and fell asleep. But not for long as she woke up demanding that someone hear her voice.

Even her yawn was short because it hurt to stretch her mouth. I held her in a romantic slow dance, pretending we were under the stars. She put her thumb in her mouth while her woob caressed her face. She scratched at her wounds. I'd paw at her hands and she'd cry out in rebuttal. Her chest looked as if it had been held captive by flames. I dressed her in the shirt made of netting from the burn unit. She hated it, but it was supposed to promote healing and decrease the risk of further opening her wounds. I had to gently rub an ointment into her skin to create a barrier and to encourage more healing. Her raw skin beneath my fingertips made me squirm for her. She was wrapped like a mummy in every failed attempt to heal her broken down skin. She took a swing at supper, but opening her mouth and swallowing made her yelp. The pain medication helped with her intake in small increments. During routine vitals they heard wheezing. My heart fell out of my chest and resembled a fish out of water on the floor. Multiple nurses were at the head of her crib, monitoring every sound. I was at the foot of her crib where I found yet another gash in her innocent skin. Upon further investigation, I found urine outside of her catheter. My head fell away from my shoulders in utter defeat. Déjà vu. I begged him out loud, "Please don't do this again!" I placed my hand on her chest. She was still breathing. "Keep breathing baby, I'm right here, I'm so sorry."

I apologized profusely. I apologized to her. I apologized to the room. I apologized to the feet under the curtain attempting to go undetected. I apologized to the window and the life outside of it. I apologized to the sky and all of spirits watching us from the clouds. I apologized with the desperation of a woman with only one thing left to lose. That is a dangerous, yet sad, disgustingly sad, woman. Dakota confessed her pain to the moon. I held her close, but she pulled away, arching her back. She bear-crawled up my torso, trying to shed her skin. Her temperature was 99.3, not a fever, but I knew where we were headed. Within the hour, she was at 100.8. Immediately, she was on antibiotics and cultures were being done. That word, *infection*, is just as lethal as the word *leukemia*. Within minutes, several people filled the room. Antibiotics and pain medications were being pumped into her. Thankfully, she fell asleep. I curled into myself and sobbed on my knees, rocking like a labeled crazy inside a white padded room. When she woke up, I attempted to give her Tylenol. The purple goop pooled inside her bottom lip. She was terrified to swallow which only meant one thing - mucositis. Even though we knew it would be coming, its arrival was still soul crushing and weakened our will to push forward. But the only way through it was through it. We had no other option but to endure the impossible to endure and march on.

With one foot in front of the other, our boots were barely on the ground. She began scratching at her chest and I noticed her dressing was falling off which was yet another risk for infection. The devil then decided to capitalize on our depleted weakness with another fever, 100.6. It took years, but she was eventually able to choke down some Tylenol. A dirty diaper with open wounds was a risk of infection. A catheter was a risk of infection. A dressing change was a risk of infection. Despite wearing masks, being sure not to breathe on her, and our hands in gloves shielding her from our touch. Just our presence in her space was a risk of infection. Everything and everyone was a threat to her life. We were battling an uphill battle, destined to lose her. I bathed her in antibacterial foam and caked her in ointment. I was throwing hail Mary's left and right, throwing every piece of myself against the wall in hopes of saving her from his constant swings at her life. Everything I did was to protect her, but it was like covering a hole with plastic while it rips at the other end. He was fighting me every step of the way. She didn't look well as she was gray in color and pale. She looked as if she were tight roping lifeless. I asked for a temperature check and she read 101.6. Battling one another, she swallowed down more Tylenol. Leaving the two of us battered and beaten, breathing heavy in our own sweaty mess. My heart was barely beating and my eyes were on fire. I longed to blanket the floor and succumb to its depths. But I couldn't sleep, not until I knew that she would wake.

The first fever was like a punch to the gut and ran away with my breath. The second one forced me to my knees. The third curled me into the fetal position while taking my heart from behind with a pair of pliers. I was desperately clinging to every one of her breaths. Intently scanning her body like a detective determined to find all of the clues. My hands were always on her chest, counting her breaths. I would squint my eyes to determine the level of her struggle. My body never stopped moving, always pacing, but stood firm. My legs twitched, tingled and became infested with fire ants. The way my pants hung on my skin felt like a lighter flame teasing my skin. Even my hair hurt, the strands like the writhing bodies of Medusa's snakes. A fuzzy blanket felt like sand paper. Minutes ticked by like hours and hours slithered like years. The culture results showed no infections. The storms we were witnessing were all chemo's wrath. My shoulder took a brief break from partnering my ears. But there was still no air in my balloon. Her temperatures were still flirting with the line. The helpless romantic in me had fingers and toes crossed that the fever had broken. Secretions were flowing like a river down the corner of her mouth. Her cry was like a whale song blanketing the ocean in the night. Her sadness was a broken no child should know and what every mother's nightmares are made of. With her warmth burning holes in my chest and her tubes cradling far too many medications in my arms. The song playing in background saying all of the words my tongue can't speak, "You'll get better soon, 'cause you have to."

The chemotherapy had stopped and with fluids, she was clearing the toxins from her body. But because she wasn't eating or drinking, she had to begin TPN again and start more medications to help her burns heal. Her catheter was out, but not without leaving its mark, requiring more wound care. At this point, she had her oncology team, the pediatric floor team, wound care, respiratory therapist, burn unit specialists and her nurses. It had to get better soon, right? I took a walk around our block which was the sidewalk that encases the perimeter of the hospital. It was a beautiful summer night. Perfect for a bon fire and a glass of wine or a cup of hot tea on the porch. A family walk in hoodies with cuddles on the couch under a big fuzzy blanket. The normal things we all take for granted. All of the things I'd give almost anything to indulge in. I fantasized about walking down a cobble stone street on a hunt for the perfect Italian restaurant, like a scene from *Eat Pray Love* in Italy. The smell of fire-grilled bread and fancy olive oil leading my nose. What it would be like to look across a wobbly table at my husband. A long-gone memory that my brain faintly remembers. A good sweat session in the gym or a run in the park. Grilling outside while the wind like a child begs for a taste. The sound of a festival with a live band outside playing under the lights of the stars. The luxury of the little things that are big things. My high roller shekels have paid top dollar for my most prized possessions. I have paid with my soul for her breath, her smile and her physical body in my arms. She is priceless and I had sold my soul to the devil for her. I had all that I could ever want and more in our before. In our now, not a second came without intense effort. Every minute was earned. But I had everything I needed and I longed only for forevermore.

I longed for forever but we only had our now. Her burns were slowly healing and she had finally been declared fever free. Her chemo had been cleared, but her mucositis was still raging in full force. She was still on TPN as she was not taking in more than a few ounces of liquid a day. She was still on morphine as it was the only way she would take anything in by mouth and find rest. The waters were far from calm, but the tsunami had passed and she was floating on the surface. Her multiple teams had decided that they would like to set a goal to get her well enough for a home visit in the next few days. They expected her numbers to crash again in the upcoming week. It was predicted that we would be admitted to control fevers and recover in order to begin chemotherapy again the following week. In order to give us this staycation from our hospital life, a few things would have to happen. Her pain would have to be managed by oxycodone rather than morphine as I could administer the oxy at home but not the morphine. She would also have to prove that she could reach the goal of 20 to 30 ounces of fluid a day to be sure she remained hydrated. If we were able to buckle down and make this happen, we would be able to be home at night. During the day we would be at clinic to receive chemotherapy, but we would be able to be together at night outside of the hospital. It was a mountain of expectation from a beaten down infant, but she knew no quit. We knew we were wading in rising waters with a hurricane brewing just a few feet ahead. A breath in between would help to give us all the strength to endure the storms coming our way. We washed our faces, wiped the sweat from our brows, put on a new pair of sweatpants and entered the batting cage.

She would take in one, maybe two ounces of liquid, water mixed with juice or Pedialyte® via syringe. But it was few and far between as the blister covered both her upper and lower lips. She was tolerating the oxycodone, not nearly as well as the morphine, but she was making do. She began to slowly take in frozen fruit, but in such small quantities that it was immeasurable. I had been making enough milk to fill an entire deep freezer which bought me a few months after diagnosis. Unfortunately, my supply was dwindling. I had stopped producing and she had not been taking much by mouth for months. We had to begin introducing formula which she was not at all a fan of. Maybe it was that her tastebuds were completely destroyed by the chemotherapy or maybe it was the bloody blisters that layered her mouth. All of which was completely validated, but did not negate her need for nutrition to not only get a break outside of the hospital but also to continue in her marathon of a fight. She refused a bottle completely as the sucking only increased her pain. She began drinking from a toddler cup and much confetti was thrown. That was a win. All the while, she was receiving a chemotherapy along with fluids that ran for a few hours. While the chemo ran, we got packed up to head home. We escaped our four walls with wagon ride, chemo pole in tow, around the halls of our floor. We were rarely outside of our room and it was beyond noticeable as she would break her neck looking into every room we passed. After hours that held no end and flushes that just came off as antagonistic, we were finally on our way home.

$\mathcal{W}$e were all in the same bed, but we were up every three hours and the morning came too quickly. I was running around like a chicken with its head cut off. I had barely used the bathroom and brushed my teeth before running out of the door. I was adorned with blood shot eyes and bags for days as we left the hospital just after supper time, getting us home around seven in the evening. It was now not even eight in the morning and were on our way back. She screamed for more than half of the car ride down. I swear she knew what was coming. Within seconds of our arrival, the chaos began. We were immediately rushed into a room for blood pressure, temperature, pulse, ox and a weight check. The urine test was on go with cotton balls inside her diaper. I was hoping for enough pee with no peeled layers of skin. Smiling kindly with good mornings, but I still hadn't had coffee. Her oncologist shined a bright flashlight inside of her mouth, showcasing the cauliflower heads. He said that her immune system was declining. His words like a giant gust of wind, challenging my balance. Stay standing, Mama. It was expected that she would spike a fever and stop eating, which meant we would be admitted. My stomach flipped like Olympic gymnasts were performing their floor routines simultaneously inside me. We had barely been home but a few hours and we were running on yesterday's adrenaline. We were placed in a private room and she was tied to a pole with tubes everywhere. She was exhausted and trying to close her eyes, but the beeping was relentless. Just as her breathing would deepen, bodies would flow in and out, a revolving door. I would pick her up and she would bury her face in my shoulder. Her tiny body grew heavy and I would ever so gently begin to place her in the pack and play. The blood pressure cuff would then squeeze her leg and she'd kick, making the numbers climb. It would restart and she would kick again, screaming at this point. The numbers would soar. She was beside herself and there was absolutely no chance of her finding rest now.

I couldn't remember the last time I had slept. The back of my head kissed my upper spine in defeat. The walls were all consuming, closing in with each passing hour. The room was like an ice box and the isolation was a visual metaphor. We were again bound by four walls, segregated and isolated. I would listen to the faint voices and smile at the laughter. The distance between us and human interaction was suffocating and my thoughts were operating on a new octave. Combine every horror scene of the girl in a dark dungeon room, clawing at what is left of her shirt as she tosses her head back screaming at the ceiling. Multiply that quantity of scenes by one thousand, and that is exactly where my head was. She had slept maybe all of 30 minutes and my arms felt as if I were holding up 30 brick houses while on roller skates. We were both hitting a wall so we took a walk. A yellow wagon with a lion on it, her chemo pole in tow. It was a delightful and disgusting sight all the same. Like biting into a dark chocolate cupcake with a lemon curd center. I would pull her in circles, lap after lap. Bumping into the corners as I am admittedly a terrible driver. In my defense, pulling a heavy wagon with a pole full of poison around tight corners is an art. I watched her calmly while taking note of the red numbers counting down. The finish line was within sight and we were both growing antsy. We would get lost in a mural on the back wall with our "wolf wolf", AKA Chiefy. We would review each one of the characters, name the objects and pretend as if we were with them, enjoying a summer night of fireworks. We were supposed to be done 20 minutes ago, but the red numbers were still showing 10 more minutes. It felt like my head was inside of a microwave. I couldn't help but stare at the pump, still three minutes to go. Time was at a stand still and we were both crawling out of our skin. We were sick of one another, sick of ourselves, just sick. With a loud beep, we were finally free. But now we had to flush. I was seconds from leaping off of the cliff, but with her eyes on me, I held on.

I packed frantically while the flush ran. It was my way of holding on. Another loud beep, cap changes, and I ran out of there with her on my hip. It was pouring out. Of course it was. The day in resemblance of my feelings. As we hit the highway, she fell asleep. I would have loved to see the back of my eyelids, but a 45-minute drive was ahead of me. As soon as we got in, Daddy took her while I melted on the floor of the shower. I curled into myself and sobbed. I begged the water to wash away my agony. I had no appetite. That was gone too. She didn't want to eat either. The night was on fast forward and we were desperate for sleep. Our desperation was met with nothing but ups and downs. Rinse and repeat. I would pace the room, bouncing, humming, and forcing my legs to hold us both up. She'd scream into my ear, drool all over my shoulder and contort her body in ways that shouldn't be humanly possible. She would rest in increments, but even her rest was restless. The alarm sounded with a dark sense of humor. It was like Groundhog Day, but a twisted version of the worst day ever. I shook my head while moving about on autopilot, thinking "how in the hell could this be our life"? This was, in fact, our life and today would be a repeat of yesterday, only longer because she needed a blood transfusion. A scream fest drive to the hospital. Followed by a swoop into a private room with test after test. Another room filled with multiple bodies and too many hands. More screaming, buckets of sweat, and exhaustion meant to deplete an army of men. Obnoxious beeping and blood pressures on the hour, every hour. My arms bouncing wet rocks while she found seconds worth of sleep while listening to my heartbeat. Wagon rides for distraction and movement outside of standing still. Taunting countdowns and incessant beeping. Watching her gray skin grow a light shade of pink was fascinating, yet gut-wrenching at the same time. Flushes that took hours and my no patience met with an angelic patience. Again, we were on our way back to the in-between. I was feeling pressured from all sides to step outside of our world. I understood the argument and the fear of my being consumed with our darkness. But the very thought of leaving her felt like death itself. Despite everything in me screaming no, I was a good girl and said yes. I took a shower with intention and not just a quiet place to lose myself. My makeup bag laughed at me and I wasn't so sure my hands would remember how to paint my face. I briefly considered an outfit that didn't consist of sweatpants, but that was short lived. When the time came, like a performer with her vocal cords severed, I choked.

I sat there in a bed that wasn't mine, sobbing and choking. Stage fright, like standing on a huge platform, the bright lights made my eyes squint. There were too many eyes on me, and with my hand on my stomach, I longed to encase myself inside my spine.

I wanted no parts of out there. Just the thought was like sucking on a sour head for four hours too long. I had an enormous amount of guilt, like the staging crew and all of their equipment crashed on top of me. I backed out like a scared little girl refusing to answer the door. My family pushed back, my friend cheered me on with poms poms and all. I felt like a torn piece of paper falling through a storm. I couldn't see, let alone hear a sound. My body was flailing and the ground was years away. I was drowning in a self-inflicted pity party, the confetti being my own downpour. After far too many hours, I put my big girl pants on and decided to go out there. The night smelled of honeysuckle, bon fires and sweet wine. The outside deck lit up with fire-filled lanterns and barn lights. I had forgotten how pretty light could be. The breath of people made my skin peel back like an orange and formed a ball behind my tonsils. I found rather quickly, that I felt more comfortable showcasing my scarlet letter rather than hiding it, both on my chest and my tongue. In the midst of sopping wet faces and broken hearts bleeding all over the plates scattered on the table, God sent an angel. A face from our world came walking towards me. I leaped out of my chair and ran to her. Like tunnel vision, I was full speed ahead towards the arrival of a long-lost hello. Embracing her felt like home. She was with me just hours ago, in our world. She was talking me through the roadblocks and grief of attempting to save my child. Now she was out here, fake smiling through the stickiness of a shared meal not served on a tray. Just like me, she was pretending to be far from our in there. The two of us making an attempt to actively participate in the "normal." Acting as if children were not dying despite our every toss at the wall to keep them alive. God shows up in the most unexpected places at the most perfect time, reminding us to still live while dying. I had been on autopilot, survival mode. I was going through the motions but I had become a disconnected version of a human. Not consciously or willingly, but an automatic change in attempts to survive. The loss after loss in such a short amount of time, had hit me like a tackle from the back at the 10-yard line. I wasn't able to see past the haze, like a concussion that has yet to return my vision. The fog was so thick, my eyes had succumbed to its inevitable layers. I had immersed myself in the fall off the cliff, embraced the crash into the tresses below. I welcomed the engulfment of flames and the kiss of death. I was dying trying to save her. On this night, there was a faint tickle in my ear, whispering hope that maybe there was a sliver of life left in me yet.

A spark had been ignited in me by venturing out there, far beyond my comfort zone. I couldn't get through the doors fast enough and my arms couldn't find her body any quicker. She was safe. She was my safety, my comfort. She slept in three-hour increments which was an improvement in comparison to the last few nights we had. We had just one more day left of chemo in clinic. It had all become pattern now and despite the fear of her crash, she was on high. She was eating cold, mushy foods and her liquid intake was still up to par. She began pulling herself to standing and walking around the playpen supported. This was a huge win as in the last few weeks, there were times she would fall into her lap while seated. It was devastating as physically she had been thriving since she was three weeks old. To watch the medications take away her abilities broke my mama heart in a way that cannot be healed. To see her physically on the move with assisted independence made my heart do flips. With all of the excitement, our day went by rather quickly and we were home in our in-between, enjoying a summer Friday night outside. She had slept much the same as the night prior, but woke in good spirits. We were admitted in the morning as it was now Saturday and clinic was closed. She was fever free, eating, drinking and receiving a few hours' worth of chemo. The hospital walls have a way of draining the mind and the body like running a marathon with little to no training. Seven hours in the hospital is like 10 weeks in the desert with 500 pounds on your back with no water. Arriving to our in-between with no gas in the tank leaves no room for conversation and absolutely zero patience for anything. There was a need to escape so desperate, mental survival was completely dependent on it, yet there was nowhere to escape to. We were completely trapped, bound by four walls in every place we took up space, and we had never been more claustrophobic.

The last few months were caving in on me and with my arms behind my back, I couldn't swim. I had endured moments that required me to readjust more often than I cared to admit. Moments where inside, I had quite literally fallen to the ground, began kicking and screaming like a toddler in the midst of a tantrum. Followed by standing with the strength of an entire army, adorned with war paint and a poker face meant to kill. All of which was necessary to get through to the next day. Hell, sometimes it was necessary to make it through the next 10 minutes and that was okay. In the normal world, I wasn't at all normal. I never was. To the eyes of those dressed in black robes with their gavel in hand, I was not handling well. Neither my emotions nor temperament were perceived with rainbows and was quite the opposite in fact. There must have been something wrong with me, but to them there has always been something wrong with me. They would insinuate that I was making it worse on myself, that I was the source of my own pain. Like a knife to my wrists, I was pushing down like butter through my flesh, choosing to bleed out. I understood, and they were not all wrong but neither was I. I wasn't okay and that was okay. In the pediatric cancer world, I was still standing, and that was a feat in and of itself. My feelings were validated and I was never on the stand under fire, taking bullets from every direction. Everything and nothing was wrong with me and that was okay. I was okay even when I wasn't and that was okay.

It was okay that I was pouring every ounce of myself into saving my daughter every single day, but that wasn't okay. Every breath I took in had become about making her as "okay" as possible, in all of the not okay. I didn't have one second to grant myself, let alone my marriage, family, friends, or what was left of any of that. The whole damn world could have been on fire and I wouldn't have blinked. It wasn't a choice, but a necessity, and I was defending myself daily. Despite the many strong grunts from the people in the back, may you forever hold your peace. I had absolutely no idea what I was doing. My feet were submerged in quick sand mixed with acid. I was drenched in gasoline, dancing with a box of matches while he held the torch to the small of my back. Nothing had taste, and insomnia became my best friend. I was actively living out my worst nightmares day in and day out. I was barely breathing and that was okay. It was on the tip of my tongue countless times to just scream, "Don't look if it bothers you!" I would ask them politely to hold tight to their banana peels, to either clap hard or go find their car. I grew deaf to their megaphones and their protesting in the street aggression. I assured them that nothing they could say would ever be louder than the voice in my own head. There was no one harder on themselves breathing than me. Every word that they had thought or had the balls to say out loud, I had already whipped myself with one thousand times over. The pole vault bar has always been set sky high, and there has never been a crash mat beneath it. I cautioned them to approach with caution or move right along and I have no regrets. I had no expectation for their comprehension. Their shoes looked nothing remotely close to mine, therefore they could never fathom my steps. If I could wrap my padded room mind around that, I had confidence in their sanity that there was hope for them too. I wasn't okay. I never would be okay, and that was okay.

Nothing was okay. The house was so quiet in the depths of the night, I could hear the wood talking. My mind released its grip and I fell like a body from the top of a building. Through a hollow tunnel of hell where demons, poltergeist and the devil's spawn are birthed, I fell past the mamas walking their breathless gray babies towards the blinding light in the sky. Their physical bodies barren and as wet as 10 oceans. The glimpse kidnapped my body, locked me in a vice, and held captive my breath. Once he shares his baby with you, entrusts you to be their protector, you would walk through fire, travel to the ends of the earth, before ever letting them go. Even in the letting go, you'd hold onto them for dear life. It is a living death to witness the death of your child. The thought alone is every attempt at suicide, with failure mocking each effort, forcing life within the longing for death. Someone had recently stated, "Families like yours make me appreciate the little things." It is a grotesque human flaw to only appreciate the very gift of life when slapped in the face with its death. There were still glimmers of human remaining deep inside me. Her every smile, like a swell of life. I guarded her with my every breath like a pack of lionesses. The grass had grown greener, giving Ireland great competition. The wagon rides were longer, soaking in every step. The swinging of swings were far too high, yet not high enough. Her blues were my sun. Watching her reminded my heart to beat. Her touch was my gasp for breath. I would watch my fellow warrior moms hand back their babies, selfishly praying I would never be forced to wear their shoes. Held captive by the darkness of the night, I tried desperately to claw my way out of the rabbit hole.

The forever rabbit hole of pediatric cancer is a darkness that I was blissfully unbeknownst to just months ago. The entire world of pediatric cancer was but a commercial to me as I was completely unaware. September is pediatric cancer awareness month and I had no awareness of its awareness until I was forced to know nothing else. I bought all of the gold glitter things I could have shipped despite never imagining I would wear gold, let alone gold glitter. I never thought my child would have cancer either, but here we were. It became impertinent to me to make all eyes aware by wearing pediatric cancer on my chest. I talked about nothing else outside of pediatric cancer to be sure their ears were ringing with awareness. I made it my absolute mission that no one could ever say that they didn't know. I was on a warpath against pediatric cancer and I held everyone to my fire. I took full responsibility in my selfish unawareness. Life sometimes leaves you no choice and slaps you in the face in order to put you exactly where you are meant to be rather than where you want to be. I still have yet to wrap my brain around the multitude of whys but I have not taken one moment of this journey without purpose. I have been hell-bent on making our story purposeful. Not for ourselves, but in hopes that someday another family will not have to live life while dying.

Children are dying because there is little to no funding for pediatric cancer, including research. Dakota and the warriors who have battled alongside her have received drugs meant for adult usage. My six-month-old baby took in medications built for grown men. If the cancer wouldn't take her, the treatment could. That was reiterated multiple times from the very beginning. It is not just during treatment that the effects of these drugs surface. It is long thereafter. Pediatric cancer and its treatment are a gift that continues to give for every day that life is lived here on earth. Four percent of government funding is granted for pediatric cancer, like spit to the face. Four pennies to every dollar is the worth of my daughter and warriors like her. Imagine if you were told your child could die and the world's cost of your child's life is four pennies. The fury you feel and the vomit in the back of your throat is what I live with daily. The gold glitter I wore on my chest had seeped through my pores and changed me from the inside out. My blood had hardened from the venom of pediatric cancer, but its color had turned a brassy shade of gold. Pediatric cancer killed who I was, but birthed who I was born to be, as it was my only way to continue living.

Living at home in the in-between, Dakota was thriving. Her food and fluid intake would increase gradually. She was much more mobile as she was not bound to a pole or held back by tubing. She had just started to find the strength to pull herself up into standing. The former physical therapist assistant in me was doing flips. Just as we were starting to catch our breath, the carpet was pulled out from under us. We went to clinic for counts where we found that Dakota was severely neutropenic and was ever so slightly running a fever. We were admitted and she was started on antifungals along with fluids immediately. That is the life of pediatric cancer. There is no room for plans as the next 10 minutes up ahead could look completely different than where you are standing in the current moment. Her fever went down with Tylenol but came back within just a little over three hours. With yet another dose of Tylenol, she was fever free and cultures were all coming back negative. Two out of three of her antibiotics had been stopped. She remained on one as she was still neutropenic despite receiving the recovery shot. We had just left the hospital last Saturday and here we were spending our in-between weekend at the hospital again. But she was exactly where she needed to be despite our mumbled grunts. She was sleeping very little in the night and the shot was causing bone pain. By Sunday afternoon, they permitted us to go home for a few days before beginning again. She was still neutropenic so I had to give her the shot at home, but at least we would get some in between before beginning again.

She was neutropenic during our first few days at home, so we would stay inside. I was giving her the Neupogen® shot to help her body recover from the chemo beating. She hated the shot and I loathed shoving the needle inside of her. But within a few days, the shot had worked its magic and her numbers were climbing. We were home working on finding standing again but still traveling to clinic for counts. The dust was never settled. There was always movement without planting our feet. Once her numbers were high enough to declare her not neutropenic, we ventured outside for some much-needed mother nature healing. The swings are her favorite still to this day. There is something about the wind in her hair and flying high up to the sky that allows her to feel free. Being outside with her allotted my breath that I otherwise held, and if only for just a few minutes, we felt "normal." We would never know normal again, but within our normal, this was the closest to "normal" we would get. Another not normal that we had adapted to was again her food issues. Her weight was declining and she hadn't grown in six months. Rightfully so and expected as she had been battling for her life. Her primary oncologist had said to me, "Whatever you can get in her, get in her. I need her to gain weight." Therefore, sometimes for breakfast she would eat chocolate pudding. Although it made the personal trainer in me cringe, our normal wasn't normal.

We were nowhere near normal, but adjusting in the best way we could to our normal. Sleep was lost no matter if we were in the hospital or somewhere in our in-between. When we could find sleep in the in-between, we slept together and as close as humanly possible. Sleeping all together became a necessity rather than just a comfort. In the hospital, the three of us were constantly forced to physically part when we needed each other the most. Therefore, in the in-between, we made certain there was no space between us, especially in the night. When we were outside of the hospital, taking up all of the space we could, we were at clinic checking counts. Her numbers had recovered. Therefore, we stopped the Neupogen® injections. This was done to gage if her body could maintain above neutropenic numbers on its own, deeming it strong enough to withstand the next round of chemotherapy. Within two days, her body had shown it was ready to fight. She began a high dose chemotherapy that was given over two days. This particular chemo was known for causing dangerously high fevers, rashes and sensitivity to light. As if we hadn't already been walking on eggshells, this caused us to quite literally twitch. Our blinds were shut and the lights were off as she wouldn't wear sunglasses. We were enduring the dark in the dark, begging the universe to keep fevers at bay.

The universe kept us on our toes as her temperatures hugged the fever line all throughout the weekend. With the poison coursing through her veins, her mobility and temperament changed rather quickly. She only wanted to be held, became sick at times, her intake decreased and she was a far cry from the baby she was just days ago. She was getting drops in her eyes in attempts to protect her vision from the chemotherapy in her blood. Once the chemo had run its course, she received another infusion that ran over time, with blood pressures every 15 minutes. This infusion was meant to help her body maintain some strength despite her depleting strength in hopes to assist in fighting off infections. After the hogtying had its fill, we were able to go back home for a few days. I was giving her the recovery shot again, knowing that her body would more than likely crash in the upcoming days. She was beyond exhausted and sleeping more than she was awake. In the before, I would have taken this as a mom win, and I wouldn't have known what to do with my allotted time. But I will never know that blissful happy mom dance when she is sleeping too much as alarm bells put me on alert. Sleeping too much could be a sign I was bound and determined not to miss. I was constantly and forever will be on guard and looking for the unseen. There was never an inch of her skin that I hadn't scanned thoroughly or a bump I hadn't investigated. Nothing was never nothing and could very well be something. It is anxiety-driven insanity that is beyond necessary to have any chance at keeping a child warrior alive.

While I was twitching with fear with the devil's pistol in my spine, standing on a stage, people were throwing banana peels. Every warrior family has a choice in the course of action with their child's diagnosis. Not only do they choose how to make an attempt at saving their child's life, but they also choose whether to do it privately or with a megaphone. I played tug of war with myself for well over one month before I stepped into my light and picked up the microphone. Vulnerability is something that quite literally forces me into a corner cowering like a battered woman. But once I got over myself and my self-loathing feelings, I realized it had absolutely nothing to do with me. I wasn't put here for myself, but for others. I had a choice - to suffer in silence as I had grown accustomed to because crying is weakness and weakness is not permitted. Or I could step outside of myself, with my shaved head and tattered pieces. I could choose to showcase my vulnerabilities, our weak moments, and our hell on earth to help others be in the know. I chose to shine the stage light on my darkness to expose pediatric cancer. I begged people to look at all of our grotesque. I pleaded with people far and wide to share every bloody, gory detail of our journey. It could be perceived that I created an audience out of vanity and greed. I still beat myself up shaking my head in wonder at how I missed my mark. I chose to strip myself down, exposing every black hole inside me. Lathered in left over chemo, blood, vomit and disgrace, I stood alone on a stage with my chin tucked into my chest. My scars were invisible to the naked eye and I know I looked like a damn fool. But I didn't do it for me. I did it for her, for them.

I had lost every part of me in a desperate hope to keep her, including my job. We gave up our home and my income. Some would say that we had no bills, which was untrue. Some also argued that her treatment was cost-free due to the help from the state, which was also not entirely true. Some of the banana peels that fell at my worn shoes were so rotten and incredibly foul, that I had no choice but to harden my heart to push through the ache. The comments came in all forms and from a multitude of mouths. Many were voices I had listened to my entire life. Their words were causing my ears to bleed and my rage to outweigh my compassion for their ignorance. I was constantly swinging my fists. There was no reprieve. I grew accustomed to defending my words, my actions, my choices, my marriage, my daughter, our family and everything about what I had become myself. I had absolutely no clue what I was doing, but I was depleting myself to do my very best every single moment of every single day, and still, it was never enough. Money is truly evil and brings out the most vile parts of people. I knew I had put this on myself and I had chosen to stand on this stage. I just didn't realize how gross humans can truly be. Despite falling on my face every few minutes from slipping on dead fruit beneath my feet, I continued to stand up and speak out. I told the disgusting truth about every piece of our pediatric cancer journey and I'll pay for it for the rest of my life, but it has been more than worth it.

My truth made people uncomfortable and forced them to ask themselves questions they otherwise would never have asked. People do not like change and they especially do not enjoy the exposure of vulnerabilities. Most swallow hard down on emotions and store them in a box out of sight; therefore, out of mind. My voice was making people's skin crawl. I apologized profusely in the beginning and long thereafter. Call it an apology tour if you will. It was never my intention to sink ships around me, quite the opposite in fact. But our new world and our story was making an impact. No good can be done without some detriment. There was, and still is, plenty of demise to go around. I have stopped apologizing as I have seen the good in all of my deemed wrong doing. There are many who throw stones, who also do not wear shoes as I do. I pity and envy their perspective all the same. What a blessing it must be to shame the broken, yet douse yourself in perfection. I am quite jealous of the ability to be so naïve. What a pity it is to be incapable of seeing vulnerability as a strength and a light despite someone's dark. I may never be forgiven for my sins by human bodies, but I have already forgiven countless times. I know that there is no comprehension for those in the unknown. Things we do understand, we cast shade on as a defense mechanism. Everyone is entitled to process and cope in their own way. There is no right or wrong way in pediatric cancer as its enormity is unfathomable, and all of it is simply wrong. I made a choice to stand on the platform and to speak loudly. Therefore, I made a choice to be ridiculed and take the beatings. The thought of a child dying is so unnatural and births an uncontrollable fury. Had I chosen silence, the fire may not have been so catastrophic and people would have been made more comfortable. My stance, combined with my words, poured like lava and the damage can never be undone. But as I stare at the ash, I am not remorseful of my path. I could have, should have, done better. But I did something and I still stand by that.

I was always standing despite my incessant crash to my knees. We went to clinic to check counts and she hadn't yet crashed. I was to be on watch for fevers, lethargy, bruising, petechiae, excessive vomiting, irritability, over-sleeping and refusal of food. Before diagnosis, all of these were signs of leukemia, but I didn't know. In treatment, all of these are signs of low numbers, which means her body is weak and cannot fight off infections. Out of treatment, all of these could be signs that leukemia has returned and round two is on deck. I wasn't on watch before because I had no idea what to watch for. Since diagnosis, I am forever on watch and always ready to swing. This has made me beyond socially awkward and with my guard always up, I have become almost unapproachable. We were venturing "out" for the first time since diagnosis. There was a talent show held just for our local warriors. We were surrounded by families just like us and people who truly understood. With my shoulders wrapped 20 times around my ears, I hesitantly walked her into a large room. My shoulders softened ever so slightly at the sight of bald children, familiar faces and gazes that required no words. We were in the company of people who wore shoes like ours and as gut-wrenching as the car crash was, it felt like home. After each child warrior performed on a stage that was only lit by their light, Dakota would walk with my assistance across the stage, adorned in the child warrior's T-shirt. At first, it felt clumsy and uncomfortable. I almost wanted to throw in the towel all due to my own shame and insecurities. But the crowd adored her and she really took center stage. She shined a light that night that burst the seams of the room. Her shiny overpowered my dark shadows and encouraged me to enjoy the light rather than endure the heavy. I had never been in a room that was so heavy and light all at the same time. A room filled with grief, ache, a never-ending pain and unimaginable trauma. Yet, there were smiles wider than the horizon and laughter that made hell grin. It was a disgustingly glorious night of realizing the hell we were living in, but living despite the death that haunted us. The universe has a way of showing us what is best as we have a tendency to not see it until it's right in front of us.

The following day was our wedding anniversary, the first one since diagnosis, and only our second one since our wedding day. Hesitantly, we attempted a meal together outside of the hospital, outside of our in-between and well outside of what was left of our comfort zone. The night was just that, uncomfortable. We were uncomfortable in our own skin. Our clothes were itchy. Our minds were speeding, yet on pause, and our lips had nothing to say and everything to say within the silence. It was an absolute miss, but at least we had attempted to swing. I was up to bat again the next morning as I was attending a fundraiser held in Dakota's honor. My hands felt like I was holding onto hot ice. They were so warm. They were swollen and the sweat could have filled buckets. I knew everyone in the room, but I felt like I was surrounded by strangers. I longed for their touch, despite holding back in the embraces, thinking about all of the germs the hug held. I participated in conversations, but I was submerged beneath a pool of water for more than 99 percent of them. The eyes on me had me scoping out every possible exit, but I stayed put for Dakota. I spoke words I don't remember, but I recall my voice shaking. I was physically there, but I was not there at all.

I was too far from where I needed to be and again the universe slapped me hard in the face with that truth. I had FaceTimed with my husband and Dakota in which I noticed some bruising on her forearm that wasn't there less than three hours ago when I was with her. Panic engulfed me in its wave and I couldn't get back to her fast enough. I was hasty in my exit and more than rude, I have no doubt. But I didn't care about letting anyone else down, as my attendance in that room that day let the one person in the world I cannot afford to let down, down. By the time I got back to her, she was more purple than she was pale. I had already alerted her team and because it was Sunday, we had no choice but to expose her to the ER. She had seven new bruises that had developed from the morning through the afternoon. Her platelets were dangerously low, so she received a transfusion. We spent our wedding anniversary in the hospital, but we were still together. We were able to go home that night and the next morning we were in clinic. Her blood was now also low, so she received a three-hour blood transfusion. We were again able to leave the hospital and I was to give her Neupogen® shots at home in hopes of helping her counts recover. We were exhausted to say the least. We had run around outside of our world for three days straight, and we couldn't help but feel as if we were paying for it. It had wiped us out physically, emotionally and mentally. No one was capable of beating us up more than we beat ourselves up, but people sure did try.

There was some question as to our choices, once again, and it most certainly would not be the last. The actions in question were our attendance at the talent show and the people around her. In some ways, I understood the questions, the confusion and my action of exposing our story publicly, therefore expecting some backlash. In other ways, I felt as if I were constantly defending us and repeating myself. But nonetheless, I stepped up to the plate and swung ever so gently, praying I didn't strike out yet again. I began by reiterating that MRD negative does not mean cancer free. MRD negative means that the body is responding to treatment so far. At any time, the body could become resistant to treatment, which would allow cancer cells to grow with vengeance. Treatment for child warriors battling leukemia could last as long as two to three years. The reasoning for this, despite how early the body attains clinical remission, is that leukemia is aggressive and therefore endurance is key. Dakota had reached clinical remission one month into treatment, but in hopes of maintaining her remission, she would remain in treatment for up to two years. In regards to the questions about the people around her, I treaded carefully. On day one of diagnosis, we had to decide right then and there who would be permitted around her. The reasoning for this was not to cut people out of our lives or to take away the right to know her or vice versa, despite popular belief. Every breath, every touch, every speck of dirt could have taken her life. Therefore, in order to keep her alive, we had to take our incredibly large circle and make it as small as humanly possible. I knew feelings would be hurt, and I would take the licks of selfish emotions. But I cared more about keeping her alive than the feelings of others, including myself.

No one and nothing would ever come before Dakota. No one and nothing ever has and no one and nothing ever will. We chose less than two hands full of people out of 70 plus, who would be permitted to be around her. We chose based off of environment and heads of families. It didn't matter what we chose, in someone's eyes, we would always have chosen wrong. But we chose as best we could in our land of little to no choices. What I did not anticipate was feeling more comfortable with others like us than those closest to us. Her medical team and families who wore our shoes understood this life in the same manner we did. This was life and death. They were as clean as we were, literally disinfecting every object before the warrior even enters the room. They were just as isolated as we were. Again, not by choice, but out of necessity. They were as cautious with breath and space as we were, yet we were capable of existing in the same space. I was surprised by my comfortability, so I shouldn't have been taken aback by the jaws on the floor and shaking heads around me. My heart is bigger than I am physically, therefore I felt the pain that I had caused by my choices without choices. I never had any intention of hurting anyone, yet I knew all to well I was inflicting pain. Looking back, I could have, should have, would have. But I wouldn't change one thing. Because she is still here, and there is testimony in that.

CHAPTER 7

I was continuing to give Dakota the Neupogen® shot to help her counts recover. She was miserable, as the longer the medication was in her system, the worse the side effects were. She didn't want to stand or sit. She only wanted to be held. At night, she howled at the moon and scaled my torso like a baby cub. Because she was an infant and had no words, I listened hard to her speaking through movement. She was enduring bone pain, which was a main side effect from the recovery drug and approaching well over one week with the injection, the pain was at a high. We went to clinic to asses how her counts were responding to the shot. In clinic, there were a few volunteers, one of whom, was a quiet, always smiling and slender man. Everything about him was incredibly kind and gentle. He would watch Dakota from a distance and sometimes build blocks with her. His presence spoke volumes, despite him being a man of few words. Before we left for clinic that morning, I had read the 30 days of stories in advocacy for pediatric cancer, through our local foundation. Like an 18-wheeler to the gut, I saw the all too familiar, kind face staring back at me, holding a picture of his son's face. He was quiet because there were no words. He was gentle because he had no fight left. He was overwhelmingly kind because his shoes looked like ours. He had lost his son to pediatric cancer just a few years before we had entered this world. At first, I couldn't fathom how he could continue to show up in the very place that his son battled for his life. But rather quickly, I understood more than I knew I understood in the moment. Returning to the place where his son fought to live was holding onto the life he lived, holding onto him. Helping other warriors smile through their battle was honoring his son's smile through the fight. Living in the space that took his son's life was his only way of continuing to live at all. I get it completely. When we walked into clinic that day, I threw my arms around him and pulled him in close. I didn't have many words either, but it was one hell of a hug. The love is different between two warrior parents because the pain is the same.

There is not a soul on this earth who understands the insanity of a warrior parent like another warrior parent. The only way to endure death while living is to release the grip of sanity and embrace insanity. I was packing for our clinic visit when the phone rang, informing me that we didn't have to go in for counts because her numbers were very high the day before. I was to stop giving the injections to see if her body could hold numbers above being neutropenic on her own. I would have to be on watch for symptoms of low blood or platelets which would indicate a crash. If she crashed, we would end up back in the hospital without moving forward with chemo. If she was able to maintain her counts, we would be admitted to the hospital for chemo. Insanity. We were just days away from her first birthday. Nothing looked like anything I had envisioned approaching the celebration of her first year of life. I couldn't throw her a pizza and ice cream party, let alone the bash she more than deserved. A local organization had reached out to me and offered to throw her a birthday party fundraiser. These people were as genuine in person as they were over the phone. They were larger than life, yet more humble than a lost soul in a dark alleyway. They had hearts big enough to heal the world and they were on a mission to do just that. They were more than willing to do something for Dakota than we couldn't dream of doing. They were filling a void we could not fill and they were doing it all out of the kindness of their hearts. From day one, they all felt like a giant hug and they have never let go.

I couldn't let go of anything. I was desperately clinging to all that I could while hoping for tomorrow. Most mamas sob at the loss of their babies as they approach the one-year mark, on the precipice of toddler life. I was balling in gratitude because we had made it this far. Some days, I longed to fast forward to year seven and cured. I was grateful for our all too brief before of breastfeeding, rolling over and finding standing. But much of her infancy had been stolen and replaced with a fight to live. I wanted her to live more than I had ever wanted anything. I was pining for her survival like the stranded out to sea thirst for water. I dreamt of seeing her fair skin without devices embedded inside, free from a chemo pole, wires and tubes. To not pierce her skin with shots and medications, a normal outside of our normal. For her to feel the tickle of grass, the warm kiss of sunshine, to bathe in dirt and pick fresh produce from a farm. To taste mother ocean's hello while specs of sand massage her feet. For her to submerge herself in a body of water, listening to the sound of quiet. Her head with hair and her face adorned with rosy cheeks. Her body healthy and thriving, pounding into a spring floor. I fantasized about her fifth birthday, then her seventh. I daydreamed about throwing the most obnoxious beach party in existence at the word "cured." I longed for her 10th birthday, then her 12th, arguing with her at 14 and 16. I had visions of her owning the stage at high school graduation. I felt the tears of me sobbing, dropping her off at college and college graduation. I could taste the tears of joy when she found her person, to see that he loves her like her daddy and I do. I felt present in the room when she would say yes to the dress. My fingers were thriving in the moment of helping her into her wedding gown, truly the most breathtaking bride. Like breath to my lungs, watching her daddy walk her down the aisle, dancing with her to our song. I was living in the words of her telling me she's pregnant and watching her bring life into this world. My only dreams were knowing she was still here and praying she gets the chance to live a beautiful life. My baby girl was turning one, and I was only hoping God would give us decades more, watching our girl grow old.

In the meantime, we were hoping for tomorrow. Her counts were good in that she didn't need to receive any blood products. However, her ANC was high, indicating a possible infection of some sort brewing. I was again on fever watch, begging the universe to allow her to be well enough to see her first birthday party. She was already fragile and now just before we would enter a smidgen of the world, it was more impertinent than ever that no one breathe on her. I was busy using my megaphone on all ears around me, both in person and virtually. I was laying the ground rules for attendance to see Dakota from afar. Taking hits of colorful names beneath many breaths, I have no doubt. I understood the perspective and I didn't blame anyone. But my concern wasn't everyone else. My only concern was Dakota and keeping her head above water. She had a lumbar puncture with chemotherapy the day before her party. This chemo was not expected to crash her body or cause mucositis. But we expected that she would feel crummy and the steroids would only amplify that. Our hopes were to have a beautiful sliver of a day, celebrating the hard work Dakota had put in to see this day.

Thankfully, the day was just that and so much more.

I got us dressed in our Dakota gear that had become our armor. I was beyond nervous, but incredibly excited at the same time. There were so many bikes lined up and I was smiling so hard my jaw ached. Everyone was in awe of Dakota, but respected her fight and maintained their distance. We rode in a truck in the procession to arrive to the party. Streets were shut down left and right for our entourage. Arriving on the property of the party was overwhelmingly beautiful. There were so many people, all dressed in orange with Dakota's name splashed on their chests. There were many familiar faces and some I didn't know. But their presence alone made me feel as if I knew them already. Dakota was supposed to ride in with her Pop Pop on his bike, but she was not feeling her best. So, I carried her in with her army all around us. It was symbolic, metaphorical and disgustingly beautiful. We had our own section to be sure Dakota was kept as safe as possible. The difficulty was that everyone wanted to touch her or just be near her. Much of the day for me was spent politely explaining our distance and maintaining that distance. There was music, an auction, food, characters, bounce houses, warriors of all kinds and lots of love. I took to the stage to thank the organization and everyone in attendance. To my left, I caught a glimpse of a few of Dakota's nurses from the hospital and I was blanketed in gratitude. There was one point when I was speaking to family, but my ears left me to find another sound. My eyes swelled and I heard Dakota's godmother yell, "Kiddos!" I ran to her and we both sobbed walking towards the music. It was a song that held a space inside both of us, encased with both grief and gratitude. A woman was painting on a piece of wood. I sat between my father and another warrior. I put my hood up to seclude myself in the moment. I was pouring oceans into the ground beneath me, completely lost in the moment. When the painter was finished, she called me up to her stage. It was a very large piece of wood with a cross carved out of it. She had painted a mermaid sitting on the edge of a cliff over the ocean. Dakota Ann was written in the sea. She gifted me with her painting and I embraced her hard, explaining the depths of the song she chose to paint this specific painting to. She cried, explaining she had no idea and that she just simply loved the song. We embraced again, even harder this time. Holding each other while pouring oceans of gratitude and grief. It was yet another moment of God showing up in our darkness, reminding us, that there is light.

It was a birthday party that made fireworks jealous. The high of its ride lasted for days. The more the buzz of the party lowered, the higher the emotions grew approaching her first birthday. I was swimming in a pool of memories of the before and reliving the moments we had endured to get to her birthday. I was choking down grief in gulps of saltwater, yet my life raft was gratitude. She was still here. She was working hard and relearning to eat without fear of pain. Simple necessities like putting food inside the mouth had become wins amongst losses. Her numbers were maintaining, she was finishing up her steroid pulse, and we were preparing for daily chemo. We were spinning in this tornado of letting go of our before, continuously taking the licks from the last six months, grateful that we made it to her first birthday and hopeful that we'd have 100 more years.

It wasn't a choice, the emotional turmoil. It was like plastic bags over our heads that we couldn't rip through despite our every attempt to make it stop. Our minds had become enemy number one. Our hearts were barely beating, yet thumping well outside of our chests. In the midst of our invisible storms, we were standing proud, throwing confetti into thin air. The night before her birthday, I couldn't help but relive the hours leading up to her arrival. I had been doing squats like it was my job because, quite literally, it was my job. My husband had gone to bed after we had take-out. I was sitting on the couch with our Chief and I stood to use the bathroom. Immediately, like a wave hit me in the gut, I was bent over at the waist. Just as quick as it came, it went.

On my walk to our bathroom, with Chief at my side, it came again. I woke my husband up to let him know and alerted my doctor. She asked me to record them and to call her back. I did as she said and found that they were two to three minutes apart within the hour. We packed and left for the hospital. When we arrived, we were told I wasn't ready yet and to walk. So, we walked the halls, literally circling laps on the hospital floor. Until my water broke on my husband's boots. I apologized profusely as they attempted to put me in a wheelchair, but I refused. Less than 12 hours later, Dakota Ann made her grand entrance into this world. She had a cowlick of strawberry blonde hair, a mermaid thumb, and gave me a look like we had known each other for centuries. She performed push ups for the nurses within seconds of her life, almost a premonition of her strength yet to come. She fed from me immediately, which had become antagonistic in comparison to the months following in which we were begging her to take a bite. She loathed sleeping in the night from day one, but gave us sunshine well beyond our hearts' content. I remembered the beginning of our before just as vividly as I recalled every moment of the last six months we had fought through to get to this day. It was an out of body experience, a nightmare and a dream. Our baby had lived to see her first birthday.

Our baby girl turned one year old. She choked down chemotherapy the morning of her first birthday. Thank you for the gift encased in poison, Cancer. In clinic, they threw her a little celebration and informed us that her blood was low. They let us go home on watch as I have no doubt my face begged them to not keep us there for a four-hour transfusion on her first birthday. She was still here. She was cranky, had no interest in food, and just wanted to be held. Her feet never touched the ground. We had a few family members, supper and ice cream. There was one moment, consisting of a laughing fit that filled the room like helium. She was still here. She was up and down all night as insomnia has its own gifts. Her temperatures were all over the place and with the rise of the sun came a trip to the ER. Cancer is the gift that keeps on giving. She received antibiotics and we were sent home. She was still here. She was beyond restless and our eyes never closed. We went back to the hospital for a blood transfusion and made our way back home. She was still here. This was not at all how I had planned her first birthday, but there is no planning in the life of pediatric cancer. Our birthday warrior girl was still here. This weekend last year, I was learning how to be a mom and attempting to give her the best days. This weekend this year, I was doing all that I could to give her tomorrow because she was still here.

We had spent every day since just before her first birthday in the hospital. Thank you, Cancer. We were admitted as her fevers were incessant and her ANC was crashing. The three of us now had a swollen red eye which indicated something viral. Then, we took a sledgehammer to the face on top of the swings we were already enduring. During her ER trip over the weekend, she was exposed to measles. She couldn't fight off a cold, let alone measles. A wave of fear washed over me and I was rolling like laundry in the under tow. All the while, fury made me foam at the mouth behind gritted teeth. I could care less if a person is purple, green or red. I don't mind one bit if a person eats Cheetos, plant based or potato milk. We are all free to live as we please, but do not put my child's life at risk. We were on day six in the hospital. The skin on my chest had been made seamless with that of her cheek. She looked like she took a hit to the face from a concrete block. Her right eye was sealed shut and was a hideous shade of purple. She was so swollen, as if her eyeball had been replaced with a softball. We were a loading circle on a map, unsure of the direction we were headed. The worry in the doctor's eyes when they spoke, forced me to stand at attention, as if a sergeant were spitting profanities in my face. I was standing post on night watch, on alert for the enemy to cross over our homeland perimeter. Red bumps would indicate that they had infiltrated. Babies battling cancer could die. Not from cancer, but because their bodies are pushed to the brink of death for a chance at life. They are worn soldiers, faced down in the wet soil, bathed in blood, with wounds inhibiting their ability to stand. They attempt to army crawl but with barely a drop of

149

air left in their lungs. Their human form succumbs to the war and they only find victory in the sky. I was selfishly crying out to the heavens life a wolf beckons the moon. Pleading for an angel to scoop my girl within her wings. Begging her magical golden dust to heal all of the boo boos and for the morning to rise with the strength to live, to fight another day.

We were battling the demons of the night, fighting to see tomorrow's rise. She was spiking fevers, struggling to see out of her swollen eye and desperate for breath. She was receiving breathing treatments because in certain positions, especially on her back, she couldn't breathe. Hearing her make those rattling noises again was one of my many doses of PTSD. She was only finding rest laying on my left shoulder. She was still receiving chemotherapy despite battling her infections, and her body was worn to put it kindly. We were all beyond exhausted and running low on adrenaline. The highs we just had were carrying us through, but falling to these lows was defeating and depleting us of energy. Her fevers were incessant and the haunting word of measles was still lingering. We were all in this tug of war between battling her cancer and fighting her infections. We, along with her team, were also attempting to wrap our brains around a few protocols and political topics that directly affected Dakota. Her body was attempting to fight leukemia and a cold while being immunocompromised. We were trying to figure out how to keep her quarantined for 28 days due to her measles exposure. The protocol stated that she would have to be isolated for 28 days. But she was battling cancer and needed treatment. We were wracking our brains on how to keep her isolated, but continuing to receive life-saving drugs all at the same time. As if we needed a cherry on this already toppling over mountain of disaster, there was a vincristine shortage. Vincristine was a chemotherapy drug that Dakota received as a part of her protocol in hopes of saving her life. A pharmaceutical company had decided to discontinue the drug. Therefore, they indirectly were choosing who would live and who would die. This was all based around money. This company glanced at images of child warriors like Dakota and only saw dollar signs, expenses. Our children were deemed too expensive and their lives were written off.

I, just like every mother in the world, was of the opinion that my daughter's life was priceless and I was throwing fireballs. I was so weak, my legs felt like Jello and I had been struggling to hold her in standing. She was battling cancer and a cold, both of which could take her life. I was feeling defeated as if I were surfing on the wing of a crashed plane, my hands and feet bound by chains and an anchor pulling me to the ocean floor. But she was also being threatened by measles and facing the possibility of not receiving one of her life-saving chemotherapy drugs. This set me ablaze and I damn near bounced off of the ocean floor, soaked in oil, burning the oceans' waves in my path of destruction. We had given up everything and everyone to keep her alive for this long. Yet, he continued to come for us in every way. We had followed every rule, living bound and isolated for months without a single bark. But the walls continued to cave in like a no-win battle. We were sinking in quicksand, kicking and screaming the whole way down. We continued barking without ceasing while choking down grains. We were bound and determined to be sure he didn't win, and he didn't. Within a few days of our firestorm, her fevers had stopped and we were able to leave the hospital on breathing treatments. We would go to clinic, isolated, to receive chemotherapy, then return home, isolated.

Isolation very quickly became second nature to us. Without notice, we grew much more accustomed to segregating ourselves rather than being socially equipped. While being closed off from the world, our eyes opened. The swelling around her eyes decreased and we were starting to see her blues again. She was receiving chemotherapy, both orally at home, and through her Broviac in clinic. We were continuing to watch for signs of measles and making every attempt not to be too angry at the world. We found our happiness in her perseverance. There had been times since diagnosis in which she would fall into her lap, unable to pick her head or torso up. Despite everything she had endured, she was walking without holding onto my hands. She was furniture-surfing and pushing baby toys across the floor. It brought tears to our eyes, watering our fires, as there was still joy in our grief. She wasn't bound to a chemo pole at home and therefore pushed through her drug induced nausea to move freely. It was disgustingly beautiful and exactly what our souls desperately needed. We were broken, beyond exhaustion and barely breathing fueled by fury. She was our glue, our energy, our breath and our calm. She was what kept us alive in our death.

We had no choice but to continue living if she was choosing to fight to live. Sometimes, living for me, meant doing completely "normal" things like going to the store. I have always been a "go

big or go home" person. Some people have labeled me
excessively dramatic. I call it passionate. To each his own. I have
always enjoyed celebrating nothing for no reason at all. It has
always been the little things that should be made the big things
in my opinion. We'd had our butts handed to us in the last week
and we were in desperate need of a pick-me-up. I was
consumed in my thoughts and breaking holes through my
padded room walls. So, I went to the grocery store to escape my
reality for a brief intermission. I hated the car ride alone
because when I looked in the back seat, she wasn't there, which
sent my head spiraling. It wasn't a choice to think those
thoughts. It just was. Because it was my very real reality.
Someday, I could look in the back seat, and she won't be there.
She may not be anywhere. She may be flying around in the sky
and I may be living out my worst nightmares here, longing for a
one-way ticket to the sky. Of course, if I spoke these words
aloud, the eyes would speak before their tongues would. It
would confirm their already formed opinions of me. So, I would
swallow down my hard truths in my alone, amplifying my lonely.

I was lost in my lonely, alone staring at candy. I was attempting
to throw glitter at the wall once again. I thought movie theater
candy, popcorn and a movie night could lift us just a smidge. A
woman approached behind me saying, "I know you are Dakota's
mom. All I have is $10, but I want to give it to you." With tears in
my eyes, I told her that she didn't have to do that. She insisted,
and we both cried. On my way to the store, where I didn't want
to be driving to the store, I was thinking about my death after
her death. I was daydreaming about being away from here and
with her up there. God truly does hear the words your mouth

never speaks. He sends angels to hold you in spaces where you are unseen. He shows us where we are supposed to be despite our inability to feel our steps on this earth. God is everywhere in our nowhere and loving us through our unlovable. The love that was poured in the grocery store that afternoon continued to shower into our night. We had a movie night, with our candy popcorn and all of the dramatics. It was a little thing that bloomed into a big thing and made the alone feel a little less lonely.

Dakota had been doing well when we first came home. But within a few days, she began refusing warm food and her temperament had changed drastically. She went from laughing, smiling and dancing to being irritable, cranky and only wanting to be held. She preferred cold foods in small quantities which indicated mouth pain. We had noticed that she was cutting new teeth and we were hopeful that there was no mucositis brewing. She would put her blanket in her mouth, bite down and pull back as hard as she could. The sound was like nails on a chalkboard and the act was violent. It terrified me and broke my heart at the same time. She was still taking food and drink mildly, despite her pain, and we were following her lead. The nights were always the worst as it seemed that was when she was the most uncomfortable. I would make attempts to sleep when she slept, but for the most part, my mind wouldn't allow it. I would find some solace in running and sweating my numbness out. Sometimes mid sweat, I would break down in tears, but I continued to run. I was a type of tired that was all new to me, yet I could never find rest. Physically draining my body and my emotions at least allowed my body stillness in the night when it was warranted. My mind was a whole other beast in itself. I have always been an overthinker and becoming a cancer mom had erased my stop button. I was the spinning arrow on the circle with never ending 500 mile per hour winds behind it. I needed breaks to continue on my go, but I wouldn't take breaks without being forced to pause.

My best friend is the most gentle, forceful push of the button, and she is always exactly what I need. She rescued me from my self-inflicted demons and made me embrace my escape, even if it was just for a few hours at most. She has never censored me or placed me in a box. Despite my white padded room and white jacket, she allowed me to be freely me. In all of my grotesque and darkness, she listened with her light and loved me harder in my too hard to love. Out in public, I couldn't help but talk about Dakota and our journey. I felt as if I owed everyone an explanation, or maybe I just selfishly longed to be heard. No matter what space I was in, I felt completely out of place. I didn't fit in anywhere and I had become a kind of awkward I myself didn't recognize. The sun's warmth always reminded be that there were still small streams of warm blood running through me, that not all of me was dead yet. That gentle kiss was like a breath I didn't know I needed, and revived a gratitude for the gift of the moment. I was sitting across from my best friend at a wooden table, outside, overlooking a stunning vineyard. It was like being washed in a wave of peace that lasted a split second, but gave me the courage to return to the war. I needed the pause so much more than I had known that I needed the pause. I needed the nonjudgment more than the two of us realized. I needed the gentle push into the sun's kiss, escaping the eyes, serpents' tongue and harsh reality so that I could rise to push back.

The push I needed to forcefully push was much more than I had anticipated. We arrived at clinic the following morning, with the intention of receiving chemotherapy and heading home. This is exactly why they inform you in the very beginning, to always have a "go bag" packed as the day never goes according to plan. They had found in clinic that Dakota was not well at all and it was much more than teething that was bringing her down. She had mucositis all throughout her digestive tract and they felt more safe admitting her in hopes of getting ahead of the storm before it got worse. The goal was to keep her as comfortable as possible and encourage her intake. We had been on the top of this slippery slope far too many times already. As a united front, we were taking all precautionary measures to keep her as high above the waves as we possibly could. All chemotherapy was put on hold to give her body a chance to heal and recover. She was on medications to control her pain and fluids to prevent dehydration. With her pain under control, she was able to find sleep and not just rest, which helped greatly in her recovery. Her temperament blossomed the following morning and we saw glimmers of the girl we love and adore shining through. Within a few days, we were able to return home with continued encouragement for intake. We would return to clinic the following week to asses her recovery in hopes of continuing forward with chemotherapy.

Leukemia has a protocol of chemotherapy, steroids and some immunotherapies nationwide. Each child is its own separate case, but the protocols are a general guideline. From day one, these outlines became our lifeline. We had to stay the course to stay ahead of her cancer. The daily chemotherapies broke her body down and many times, left her struggling to stand. But that meant the chemo was doing exactly what it was supposed to do, which was to destroy all of the cancer cells in her bone marrow, reprogram the cells, and ultimately stop her body from creating cancer cells. If her cancer cells were resistant to the chemotherapy protocol we were following, she would need more invasive treatments in attempts to save her life. Bone marrow transplant and CAR-T can be fatal in and of themselves. Dakota's body was responding well to the infantile protocol she was on. However, at times, the treatment was too much. The kick while she was down was keeping her down and not giving her enough time to stand on her feet. Her team decided that they would change the course slightly in order to decrease her severe crashes. Her dips were delaying treatment and it was impertinent that we stay on schedule to be sure not to leave a door open for cancer to grow. This made our heads spin as my husband and I are beyond type A and OCD. We always have had a plan for our plans, and this was like lighting tomorrow on fire for us. We asked far too many questions as we were living and dying by their protocols. But they had kept her breathing this long, and we trusted that they were always doing right by Dakota. We stopped giving Dakota daily chemo, she skipped methotrexate, and we went right into vincristine with a steroid pulse in hopes of bypassing a crash and getting back on track.

We were navigating our new course, but cancer gets a thrill out of throwing us off course. She woke up one morning with those terrifying purple dots on her face, petechiae. Something is never nothing and nothing will always be something. We immediately rushed to clinic for counts. Her numbers were in good standing, but after an overview of her body, they found an injury to her bottom. It was more than likely caused by the prior mucositis along with antibiotics. The medications used to treat infections can cause an increase in loose bowels and mucositis is painful, so pushing to relieve pressure is natural. We were able to go home with some tools and medications to help her heal and manage her pain. It was her first Halloween. We hadn't slept as she was still in pain. We still dressed to celebrate, throwing glitter at the wall. In clinic, she received chemotherapy and took pictures with her medical team who were dressed and throwing glitter at the wall as well. At home, she began her steroid pulse and she trick-or-treated in the house. It was yet another holiday spent making do with what we had and being grateful that she was still here.

We were grateful, but we were in fact struggling. We were six months in to our new version of hell and there were still multiple marathons up ahead. It was endurance, not a sprint. In the beginning, everyone rushes in like a mob. It is overwhelming to say the least. There are so many bodies and voices that it often feels like attempting to move through a crowd at an outdoor summer concert. But the bodies lessen, the voices fade, the opinions get louder from a distance, the loneliness becomes suffocating and true colors never shine more bright. Often people have said that they don't know what to say, so they say nothing at all. The silence is so much more detrimental than that of the words actually spoken. I would spend so much time writing out an intricate, detailed update via text message, only to receive crickets back. The no sound was deafening and left holes in me that will never fill. I understand in that their lives had to continue on despite ours stopping on the dime. The quiet instilled lessens I had to learn and I will never forget. I cannot expect from others what I am not willing to put out. Every person is entitled to cope in their own manner. People run from what they cannot understand. Out of sight, out of mind is the easiest way out. The darkness of tragedy shines light on what otherwise would be cast out by shadows. Distance does not always make the heart grow fonder. In some cases, distance amplifies distance. All of the negative opinions people had of you before your world blew up, intensify in the aftermath. People are sheep and fear the roar of a lion, and sometimes the lion just needs a sheep's hug. None of it was okay, but it was okay.

Life doesn't stop with a diagnosis and we were forced more times than I care to recall, to swallow that. The worlds become segregated almost immediately and there is minimal crossover. I had unwillingly made a choice not by choice, to live solely in this world with her. My world was enormously overwhelming in that just the buzz of a fly tapping the window sent me over the edge. I had no vacancy or the capacity to take in any other parts of the other world, including other people's lives. I have no doubt there are colorful words for these statements and they are not untrue. But I stand by the statement, you don't know until you walk a day in my shoes. I promise you, most wouldn't last five minutes. I don't say that in an egotistical manner. I speak matter-of-factly. The pediatric cancer world is meant to cause a broken without healing and an unfixable destruction. It is built to take everything and everyone away with no intentions of ever getting any of it back because there is no going back. Its absolute purpose is death and with or without breath left, it will succeed. In spite of its death, we went on living. My husband and I assumed roles without choosing our roles. I took care of our inside and he handled our outside. It had been said numerous times, that he could not live in my world as I could not exist in his. He could not fix this. Therefore, he felt no purpose outside of providing and tending to the things he could control. I could not focus on anything or anyone other than her and keeping her alive. Therefore, I lived beside her 'round the clock and he kept our heads above water by dealing with the out there. He tended to things that continued on outside of our pause. He was alone in his handling, but he handled. We didn't know then that much of our handling left no space for processing the actions we were taking. There is no processing when in survival mode. There is only handle and get through the next few minutes. The space between us, our worlds, others and within ourselves was thickening with every passing second. We were as thick as thieves.

The thick vines that were ever growing, surely separated us from things and people, including one another. But on other paths, those very same vines, wove us together in a way that is unbreakable. There had been physical distance between us as my husband had to tend to outside world things, but we managed, and he was back home. Dakota and I had been pushing through her treatment-induced injury and navigating our new normal. As a newborn, she loved water. We would bathe together often, and it was a time of day we both looked forward to. After diagnosis, a bath was one of the things that we lost. Her new hardware and risks of infections took that time away from us. Her nurses helped me with some new tools to possibly gain bath time back. Her Broviac, including the tubing, could never touch water. It was literally a hole in her chest covered by bandages. If anything got wet, the risk of infection would be sky high and could send us down dark holes with no pathway back. We used aqua guard, which is a large plastic sheet with adhesive along its edges. A word to the wise, the adhesive it is adorned with is not nearly enough to lay flat on skin, especially a mobile infant. Therefore, we used a plethora of medical tape to adhere the sheet over both her dressing and all of her tubing. It was a process, to say the least. We were both a sweaty mess before I even placed her in the tub. But her joy in the tub was more than worth every second of the hassle. She didn't get to do much, so the little things she was able to do were huge. It was extremely nerve-racking for me, in that every splash she made, made me hold my breath. I was petrified that her Broviac would get wet, which meant we would have to go the hospital. She could have ended up with an infection which meant she could die. Everything could cause her death. But I was attempting in every way possible that I could, to let her live. So, she took a bath.

Bath time was successful, but the consequences showed on her skin. She was at the end of a steroid pulse at the time. Steroids came with a slew of side effects for Dakota. She very quickly became irritable, miserable, and her skin was red with fury. She was hungry, but would throw up if she ate, and sleep was nonexistent, despite her exhaustion. The bath seemed to give her a happiness, but her skin would look as if she had been sun bathing with baby oil on, no matter how lukewarm the water. Her hunger came with vengeance, but she knew if she ate, she would throw up, so she refused food. She would become well beyond the point of tired, but her legs were restless and that was just what I could see. I cannot begin to fathom what she was feeling on the inside. When I say we hadn't slept in months that led to years, I am speaking about intervals of sleep in barely a few minutes at a time. Sometimes the intervals were 20 to 30 minutes. If we were lucky, we would barely scratch the surface of an hour. Other times, we were up throughout the night, on the hour, every hour. It was grueling and left no space for tolerance of the day, but we had no other option but to power through. We made the best of the moments we had, and we tolerated even the bad ones because she was still here.

She was still here and on the move despite her spending the last six months tied to a pole, more than free as a bird. With chemo coursing through her blood, she had taught herself how to get from point A to point B by this quite original scoot. It resembled a gremlin maneuver of sorts, as her left leg would lunge her forward while her bottom ever so slightly lifted off of the floor, and her right leg stayed bent beneath her. It was creepily hysterical and draped our hearts in pride as she was moving in spite of everything meant to hold her down. After she had finished her steroid pulse, we went to clinic to begin chemo. Her blood was low, so she received another transfusion and chemo through her Broviac. She had a slight fever, but her ANC was high enough to fight off infections, so we were sent home with oral chemo daily. She was teething rather hard on top of everything else her body was enduring, and Daddy had to put in night work to keep us floating. The days were long and the nights were even longer. Her fevers were staying at bay, but between her laughs, she was miserable. Somewhere in the bitter beginning of November, she began to blossom. She had white blonde peach fuzz sprouting on her bald head, the slightest sign of eyebrows coming, and she was on the precipice of gaining eyelashes. It was only November, but we celebrated anyway. We dove right into Christmas with baking cookies, hot cocoa, Christmas music and all of the Christmas movies. Dakota ate it all up and loved every minute of it. We didn't have much, but there were moments in our before when I would have given anything to be at home with her watching Christmas Hallmark movies. Being granted this wish in this manner was not at all how I would have ever envisioned, but nonetheless, I was grateful.

CHAPTER 8

$\mathcal{W}$e were grateful for where we were, grateful we were not where we had been, but there were still boulders in front of us. Dakota's blood and platelets were in good standing, but her ANC was low. Therefore, her body was unable to fight off infections. She was finally free from isolation due to the measles exposure, but because her body was in such a fragile state, we were to remain in isolation. During these times, it was imperative that every surface Dakota could touch was sanitized to the nth degree to decrease risk of infection. Every environment we took up space in wreaked of chemicals in hopes of warding off any every day demons that could become a threat to her. The birthing of becoming a hypochondriac is inevitable as it becomes the only chance at survival for your child. Your breath alone could be a threat to your child's life, let alone someone else's. The organisms that are unseen living freely on surfaces are a threat, and it is impertinent that even the unseen be killed off to possibly keep your child alive. It is mentally draining and chips away at the human soul piece-by-piece. The tongue grows weary of explaining the unexplainable, and the mind drifts deeper and deeper into insanity. It is an inescapable mind fog that walks a fine line between living and succumbing to one's own death. With her each breath, we threw glitter at the wall, smiling through our beyond tired. We were engulfed in guilt at our own pity as her physical anguish was no doubt far worse than our own. It was a sick parallel in that her will to live fighting off her death was our lifeline. We didn't have much to hold onto, but we held tight to one another.

In the moments in which we had nothing to hold onto outside of one another, we held onto the things that lifted us. In our in-between, we had a room we slept in and a room we used like a living room. It wasn't even Thanksgiving yet, but we decided that we needed some light. So, we decorated our little living area for Christmas and put a small tree in the room we slept in. It was difficult in that much of our stuff was still packed away in storage. It was hard in that it was only her second Christmas here on earth, yet we remained grateful. Despite the grief we were working through, we forged on and brought light to our dark. Our bodies were tired from the constant up and down. Our minds and our hearts had nothing left to give. Until she sat at the bottom of the tree and looked up at the angel. There is a magic that exists in a child beside a lit Christmas tree. There is an unexplainable sliver of heaven witnessing a child fighting for their life, looking up at an angel. In that moment, once again, she breathed life back into both of us.

Despite our every attempt at light, our darkness was a force always on our heels. Dakota was phlegmy with a hive-like rash on her back and her belly. She also had a chemo burn on her bottom. Her team was aware of her condition at home. I had learned that chemo rash was quite common and I was lathering her in every suggestion I could to help give ease to her skin. She was clawing at her back, her belly and "down there". As any mother would, I was going off the deep end in search of how to help her through her pain. We were putting poison in, so naturally, poison was coming out. The diaper was becoming a breeding ground for infection and therefore a threat to her life. Common sense says, get rid of the diaper, but she was barely one year old. I bought a toddler potty and we began training. Some would say I pushed her too early, just as I did with her

165

schooling, in attempts to get ahead of chemo brain. I can't say that I myself would not have the same judgement had I been on the other side of the lawn. From where I was standing, I was just a mom attempting to decrease the pain my child had no other option than to endure. Dakota took the potty rather well. She laughed and smiled in fact, especially at the flushing. By day two of sitting on the potty, she was going. It was not just a win in that our one-year-old was using the potty. It was a win in that our baby would have less burns from chemotherapy on her skin. It wasn't at all normal, but it was our normal.

Our normal was far from normal and we were constantly adjusting our normal daily. All we had known in the last six months was possible death, poisonous chemotherapy, hospital life and isolation. The tides were turning once again and our team was preparing us again for another new normal. We were approaching the maintenance phase of treatment. This was the last phase in her treatment protocol. This phase consisted of some brief admissions and clinic visits, but the goal was to have more time outside of the hospital. She would still have lumbar punctures, intravenous chemotherapies, blood draws and IV medications. The hope was to transition to less frequent hospital necessities and more at-home medications. Eventually, she would receive chemotherapy daily at home, weekly steroids and monthly clinic visits. Transfusions for blood or platelets and antibody infusions would be based on her counts, what her body would indicate was required. This was all overwhelmingly exciting in that it gave us hope for an end in sight. It was equally terrifying in that daily chemotherapy would wear down her already worn body. As much as we had loathed hospital stays, they had become our safety net, and we felt most comfortable there than anywhere. We were cautiously happy to move forward into the next phase, but we had taught ourselves to no longer get our hopes up.

No matter how lost our hope, hope always found us. I had taken a mama breather and gone out to purchase Dakota some Christmas clothes. I was struggling in that the tiny clothes reminded me of all that we had been robbed of these last few months. I was grieving the baby who never got to wear all of these pretty clothes. Materialistic and selfish, I am more than aware. My heart never stopped finding gratitude that she was, in fact, still here. But at times, the human version of me got the best of me. I was caught somewhere between mourning the baby I had lost, and celebrating the baby I still had. God sent me yet another angel right then and there. I was standing in line to pay for the glittery Christmas outfits that I had hoped would bring light to the Children's Cancer and Infusion center. A beautiful woman in front of me turned to me and said that she knew exactly who I was. That she had been following Dakota's story and praying for us every single day. She had paid for our clothes and with tears in everyone's eyes, the grace of God engulfed all human life in the store. It was times like these that restored my faith. I was angry at God more often than not. I truly struggled every minute of every day to show Him love as I watched my baby endure horrific pain. But He reminded me time and time again, that He was still walking with me, despite my pushing Him away. When we were barely holding on, He sent his angels down to lift us up.

The war between the devil and God's angels is forever raging on.

When I got home that night after a visit from an angel sent from above, Dakota's Broviac line was not flushing. I made her team aware, and we went to the emergency room. They were able to flush her line and we were sent home. The following day was Thanksgiving Eve. There was more than enough to be grateful for. First and foremost, we were grateful for Dakota still being here on earth. We were grateful for the outpour of love and support from our community. So much had changed drastically in just a few short months. Isolation had become second nature and our loved one's lives had forged on, rightfully so. It was bitter sweet but it was lathered in gratitude. We were grateful not only for the long-lost loves, but that our loved ones were able to live happily. Despite our despair, we had one happy that was quite literally all that we needed. Dakota was still here. There were many things we had longed for, but none of them came anywhere near measuring up to our desperate need of her. We had Dakota and therefore, nothing else mattered. We had all that we needed, and we were beyond grateful.

It was Thanksgiving and we were surrounded by family, food and gratitude. I was flushing her line by pushing heparin through the tubes hanging out of her chest. She was squirming on the carpet at my knees, almost in preparation for the saltwater taste she'd get in her mouth with every flush. My eyebrows kissed my hairline and my eyes bulged out of my head as the clear liquid shot through a pin hole in the tubing. I felt the resistance, like blowing water through a sealed straw. The white tube ballooned and I immediately stopped everything. I interrupted her oncologist's holiday, taking him away from his family with my panic. He made a few calls, but the one we needed to help us through this new hurdle was not available as it was indeed a holiday. I was told to seal her tubing and dressing area as much as physically possible to block out all risks. This tiny hole was now a gateway welcome party for every life threat to infiltrate and take her away. The swarm of love downstairs was now a pool of death threats and my skin was crawling with fire ants. I had no other option but to get her through the night without allowing any monsters to find the open door. I had to get her to see tomorrow in hopes of making it all better again. I stood no chance at making anything all better, but I had learned to make our version of all better as all better as possible.

We, at lightning speed, went from immersing ourselves in family love to complete isolation yet again. The doors were shut and with eyes wide open, I spent the night swinging my sword while she slept. We had made it through the night without demons taking her away. We drove to the hospital first thing in the morning and her team, including a specialist, went right to work. I helped her nurses hold her down on a cold table. There was a woman who used things that resembled a popsicle stick and glue, in attempts to fix the tubing hanging out of my baby's chest. I was biting down so hard my teeth were grinding against each other. Sweat dripped from my brow as if I'd been running for hours. Our eyes spoke the inappropriate words dancing on the tips of our tongues. Dakota was screaming bloody murder and writhing as if she were entangled in barbed wire. There was not much kindness or compassion coming from the stranger at our table. Through masked faces with soft eyes, our angels assured me in my not okay that she would be okay. The woman was attempting to put toothpicks under the broken tubing. But the rubber tubing was a slip and slide from the combination of sweat and antibacterial solution. She used words that insinuated that Dakota was at fault for the failed attempts. It was Dakota alone who kept me bound and gagged from unleashing my motherly wrath. After what felt like endless days of interrogation, surgery became our best option.

Surgery would entail reopening her scars from her second Broviac placement on the right side of her chest and sealing them again. They would then slice open her original scars on the left side of her chest from her very first Broviac placement. A port, which resembles two bottle caps upside down, inside of her chest. They would then create new seams on her baby skin, sealing her for a third time. There would no longer be any tubing originating from inside of her and hanging outside of her. With the touch of fingertips, her port would be felt, but it would be unseen. Her skin would now be punctured with a rather large needle to administer medications and draw blood. She would now be permitted to take baths without dressings, but "accessing" her for medical necessity birthed an entirely new version of nightmares. My whole body was restless, tingly and itching with spiders being born beneath my skin. My hands were wet as if I were preparing to give a speech in front of thousands. My lower back throbbed from the weight of the world and my shoulders ached from the endless fetal position. Carrying 100-pound sand bags up mountains barefoot would be a cake walk in comparison to the hits I was taking.

The hits continued hitting. There was little to no time between her hog tying on the metal table to her head falling away from her neck, gifted by anesthesia. I kissed her forehead and demanded that she come back to me in the softest whisper. Once again, I watched her leave my sight in the arms of angels adorned in shower caps. The walls became too beige, taunting me like school girls on a playground. The deafening quiet grew louder and louder. My stomach started to turn, like a worm being wrapped around a hook. I was pacing with the speed a New Yorker at eight a.m. on a Monday. My name was called. My husband and I flew like a jet to the desk. Just the two of us were in a room that was far too white. He mentioned how quiet it was. It's uncomfortable when you can hear one another think and we both win trophies with our awkwardness. It was louder than a concert in our heads, but the room held no sound. The sound of one another's breath reminded us both how very dead we truly were. Finally, the surgeon came in, reassuring us both with her smile she was still here. My shoulders lowered a hair and I may have even cracked a smile. We walked without holding hands down hallways that I believe resemble the halls of hell. Déjà vu. Our baby blanketed in tubes and wires, painted orange. A new device proudly showing its face under her infant skin. I picked her up, embracing all of her - new, old and everything in between. She was still here and this is what we were thankful for.

She was still here, which meant we were still in the fight. Despite surgery that morning, she started chemotherapy early that afternoon. She was exhausted and irritable. Rightfully so. She had just been sliced open at the start of the day and she was now being pumped with poison and fluids. She had some sickness, which was expected as her tiny body was full to the max. Eventually, she crashed, but it was short lived as her body was so uncomfortable, it couldn't find rest. We were in the hospital, battling our demons throughout the night. Her nurses were more than accommodating and went to the nth degree in attempts to make Dakota as comfortable as physically possible. Our eyes hadn't closed, and yet the sun was on the rise. With its good morning, came more chemo and fluids. Our only saving grace at this point, was that it was likely we would be able to go home that evening. We were clinging to the hope of walls outside of these walls to get us through the bricks that were piling on top of us. Brick by brick, we made it home. We would sleep in the same bed that night and head back to the hospital in the morning.

The morning brought a winter wonderland. We were driving through the white fluffy glitter, pretending to be unrealistically normal. She had cotton balls in her diaper to assess her hydration in order to permit her receiving chemo upon arrival. Completely normal in our normal. The cotton balls flashed a green light to go, and within minutes, she was being pumped full of the devil's juice with blood pressures running every 15 minutes. Blood pressures were Dakota's kryptonite. She loathed the constriction, the squeezing and even more so, the requirement of remaining still. It would take at least three people to get a decent reading for blood pressures. I would be holding her, using my legs and arms to hold her down as much as possible. Another person would be attempting to keep her arms and legs from flailing, which only made the numbers climb. Another person would be singing or playing a movie in attempts to decrease her screaming, which again, only made the numbers soar. The other person would be battling the machine and Dakota in hopes of getting a good reading and putting an end to the madness. This chaotic scene was played out every 15 minutes. The duration was an hour at the start of chemo and another hour towards the end of the chemo running. We would arrive by eight in the morning and we would close clinic down, leaving just before or sometimes after four in the early evening. We would leave our team worn and sweaty and embark on our just under an hour ride home. I would make multiple failed attempts at getting her to eat something substantial. She was usually feeling too nauseous despite anti-nausea medications and/or too tired to even look at food. She would fall asleep in my arms, but the moment I would sit or lay back, she would scream out in protest. She would find rest in the nook of my left collarbone for 30 minutes to an hour while I bounced and paced for hours on end. Before we knew it, the morning would come without an end to the night. Like Groundhog Day, we would rinse and repeat from the day prior and continue déjà vu through the end of the week.

By the end of the week, it felt as if a year had passed. I spoke with her team, as we believed in emotional strength just as much as physical strength, and they agreed. We ventured out to a secluded Christmas tree farm for some normalcy. We were outside and the two of us steered clear of people. Instead, we allowed our eyes to grow big at the beautiful greenery. Once again, nature's beauty was no match for Dakota's. The sun, ever so gently, kissed her skin. I swear she was glistening from the inside out. Like vampires in sunlight lighting up like a disco ball, the oxymoron of light in the dark is captivating. The air was crisp, but our breath was like a warm cookie right out the oven. It was a moment of gratitude that brought swells to my eyes and forced me to my knees. We had endured many moments in the months prior that made us question if we would ever see moments such as this. To officially arrive to a place that you were not sure you would ever see is a feat as large as climbing Mount Everest and claiming a world record, all in the same day. It was a slice of Heaven I feared biting into, as Heaven had been far too close for comfort as of late. I indulged nonetheless, as the temptation was overpowering and she was my weakness. I soaked in her shiny as I once soaked in hot lavender bubble baths. I savored her like a sliver of decadent chocolate. I hit the pause button for what I wish would have been 10 plus years. I didn't want to move. Moving would catapult us into our war that for, less than a second, had separated us from it. I didn't want to go back. I didn't want to take a step. I longed to stay right there. I wanted to remain in our gift of Christmas trees, sparkling faces and warmed hearts. I showered the universe with gratitude and selfishly begged for just a few moments more.

Cancer doesn't care about your desire for moments, and spits at gratitude. Her numbers were dropping, despite my giving her the recovery shot, and her bottom was an awful shade of red. I am just as stubborn as cancer, if not more. I spit back at his nastiness. I checked in with her team and they allotted us a visit with Santa Claus with some rules in place to maintain her safety. Santa and his elves were accommodating and had much compassion towards our situation. Dakota was not a fan of the jolly old man, especially if I was not at her side. Many of the pictures were of her screaming, with the exception of maybe one or two. Still, the moment was celebrated. The following day, we went to clinic where we had found she was neutropenic, but did not require any transfusions at the time. We were to continue giving her the recovery shot and return early the following week for counts. We made the best of our weekend with our unknown up ahead. We took her to see Christmas lights, but we remained inside of our car. We were constantly throwing glitter at the wall, in attempts to give her beautiful days all while hoping to keep her alive. It was an exhausting and debilitating tug of war. Our job was to give her an incredible life all while giving her life to live. We didn't know how many days she would have here on earth; therefore, we were sure to go big for her every day.

We were granted another day when we went to clinic and found her numbers were well enough to stop using the recovery shot. It was expected that her numbers may fall, but we were hopeful that she wouldn't bottom out as she was to have another lumbar puncture followed by steroids at the start of the following week. Christmas was approaching fast and there was flour to be flung. We spent our days outside of the hospital baking cookies, dancing to Christmas carols and watching every Christmas movie we could get our chocolate-covered hands on. The week of Christmas had arrived and I was overwhelmed with emotion. This was, by far, the most incredible Christmas I had experienced in my 30 plus years of life up to this point. There were more moments than I cared to remember when I wasn't sure she would be here for Christmas, yet here she was. Her only Christmas before this, I was a working mom pulling 12-hour days. I distinctly remember being at work watching the snow fall the year prior, yearning to be snuggled up at home with Dakota under a blanket watching Christmas movies. I, in no way, ever imagined that the following year, she would have cancer and I would have been granted my wish in the most vile backwards way. I loathed our life and I was full of piss and vinegar. But my heart was incredibly grateful to not only be home with her not missing a moment of this Christmas, but that she was in fact alive this Christmas. She was not only our greatest gift under the tree, she was the only gift we even wanted and needed.

Cancer is the gift that keeps on giving. We went to clinic to have a lumbar puncture with chemotherapy injected into her spine. For every lumbar puncture prior to this, Dakota was given ketamine and versed. The anesthesiologist wanted to begin weaning her from the ketamine as she had received it countless times in the last eight months and they were weary of its long-term effects. The anesthesiologist decided to substitute the ketamine with fentanyl. With my jaw on the floor as I had thought morphine was loaded enough, my blood ran cold at the thought of my baby on fentanyl. I was told she would be fine and that this was much better for her. It was insisted that this combination may even keep her more relaxed throughout the entire procedure. Dakota had other plans and literally blew everything that was said completely out of the water. She woke up mid procedure like a bear. She sat straight up and it took multiple adults to get her onto her back again. The bear-like characteristics continued on long after she came out of sedation. She was angry, bright red, aggressive and on a war path, as was I. We were both filled with fury and our skin was speaking the words our lips couldn't possibly speak out loud.

The message was received and I was told ketamine would be used next time rather than the fentanyl. We topped off her anger with a dose of steroids caked in chocolate pudding. Dexamethasone tastes and smells like rubbing alcohol. Chocolate is the only thing I had found to mask most of its nose-turning properties. This spoonful of chocolate was not the calming wave of peace that comes with most chocolate. This hellish chocolate would birth a monster in any sane human being and leave an ash-filled forest in its path of destruction. It was a rough day, but even worse days were already on the way.

Nothing looked remotely close to what we had hoped for, but were both still here. I knew because he got a haircut. I had showered and put on something other than a leukemia shirt. We still wanted to look good for one another. Effort equals a win. The car ride filled the air with words that were meaningless, surface level and singular. It was stiff like a board room full of lawyers. The Christmas music made a failed attempt at lending a hand. There was a view of the outside world, but it was a world we didn't exist in anymore. A fire was lit under his seat, and he spontaneously changed our plans. He drove us to an environment completely out of both of our comfort zones. It was noisy, chaotic and there were far too many people. Ironically, this box was necessary for the two of us to be alone together. It was overwhelming to put it gently, like a frenzy of great whites thrashing around me. It was a blatant slap across my face of just how hermit-esque I had become in my no other option isolation. This random spot the two us would have never entertained was surprisingly working its magic, distracting us from one another. We became lost in the crowd as our distance only grew thicker. He was in one place and I was in another. We were still in one other's sights, but we were nowhere near close enough to actually connect. We both wanted to, but we had forgotten how to be human. I have no control over an itch and I chose to call out the giant elephant hovering heavily above us. As expected, he retracted like a broken bungee cord. I bubbled over like a hot pot of pasta, white foam and all. We discussed things no two people should ever live to discuss. Our eyes couldn't find one another and there once was a time we would lose ourselves in our gaze. Despite our hearts bleeding all over the table, there were no words left to speak. The only options left were to continue on or call it. Only because the two of us refuse to fail at anything, we continued on. Somewhere between that awkward walk from one table to the next, the air shifted. The space decreased and he wasn't sitting across from me. He chose to sit beside me. His arm found my shoulder and his lips made a pass at mine. My head found his chest like the pillow I thought I had lost. We smiled in unison and at times we even shared a laugh. I had forgotten that sound. As the fudge dripped romantically down the edge of the cake, my heart melted for him. We left the room meant to increase our distance, closer than we could have ever imagined. His hand found mine as I held on desperately in fear of losing the grip again. Nothing looked remotely close to what we had hoped for, but we were still here.

We were together for Christmas. We spent Christmas with our baby who was battling cancer and enduring side effects from steroids, but she was still here. We were home for the holidays, surrounded by friends and family and not at the hospital.

Dakota had moments of pure joy, but also many moments of pure misery. Through no fault of her own, steroids induced a shade of Jekyll and Hyde like nothing I had ever seen. This Christmas was entirely different from any other Christmas we had known, but as a family, we made do. It was lit up with light, love and gratitude. There was a plethora of cookies, food and hugs, all of the things needed to lift the soul. There were elephants and spaces that couldn't be filled. But everyone bit down and smiled hard because it had nothing to do with us. It was bittersweet to say the least. There was far too much to say, yet not many words were spoken. The children were happy and Dakota was breathing so nothing else mattered much. We said our goodbyes and people went back to living their lives. We returned to our isolation with full bellies and longing hearts, but nonetheless, we were grateful.

The night challenged our grateful hearts with broken ones. Dakota was having exorcism-like episodes. She would be wrapped up in blanket in one of our laps, more than content. Then, like a bee sting, she would scream a scream that made mirrors shatter. Her back would arch as if a demon were attempting to escape from deep inside her. Her body would thrash like a great white on a hook. There is no pain like seeing your baby in pain and there is nothing you can do to make it stop. It didn't matter if she was held in standing or sitting, the demons were attempting to throw her out of our arms. It didn't matter if music was playing or if we were slow dancing in complete silence. The monsters were forcing their way up her esophagus. At times she would pass out from exhaustion, but it wasn't restful and it was short lived. Cancer and poison were quite literally holding her body hostage and even with her in our arms, we were unable to set her free. Our eyes never closed. Our bodies never found stillness, but the morning came anyway. To our surprise, with the rise of the sun, her demons had released. She woke up smiling her soul-healing smile and clapping her hands as if to the mock the hell of the night. The night had never slept, but the day was ready to play.

During the day, I took two hits to the stomach that took my breath away. Her bald head had finally grown some white peach fuzz. Her eyebrows were visible in sunlight and her eyelashes were giving her gorgeous blues some definition. But cancer gets his kicks by destroying beauty with his ugly. I rubbed my hand on her head in a caressing way, just as any other mother does. I felt the nest in my hand and the lump in my throat rose immediately. I was terrified to flip my hand over, knowing damn well what was lodged in its palm. With vomit holding captive my breath and my lips pursed to hold it all back, I rotated my hand. The visual of what I already knew gutted me and left me hanging from nothing in a barren desert with my insides outside. Her strands of newly grown hair in my hand were melting the flesh from my palm. It was like watching all of our hopes written on paper set fire and its ashes taken in the wind of a tornado. Despite the drippings of my neck creating a puddle of blood beneath my knees, I smiled for her as she clapped her hands, completely unaware that our world was some twisted nonfiction written by the devil himself. As if my bleeding out in front of her in this moment weren't enough, she stood with her cart to make her way to her kitchen. As she pushed, her left leg was dragging behind her. It looked like a tree trunk being pulled by a metal chain. There was no bend in her knee, no point in her toes and no lift from her hip. It was cancer's dead weight just trailing behind the rest of her body. I sat there, already dead and unable to blink. There was no unseeing what I had just witnessed. I was stunned and paralyzed as I couldn't move or even speak. Yet every inch of me felt as if I were already miles up the road sprinting to nowhere while antagonizing the sky with my screams, demanding that they hear me.

I felt as if no one could see me, let alone hear me. I felt completely alone, falling down a rabbit hole lathered in darkness with sound proof walls. My hands were bound, kissing my spine, and my legs had been shattered with no bones left to break. Every piece of me was held captive in his grip, except for my eyes, to be sure I could witness the slow, painful death he was inflicting on my baby. I had been a personal trainer and a physical therapist assistant in our former life. Strength was my middle name. Yet, I was unable to heal, let alone rehabilitate my infant daughter to her full potential as I was the very reason, she was so debilitated. Steroids are known to cause joint pain and deterioration. I was pumping them into chocolate pudding and spoon-feeding it to her with coos and praise. I was the queen of Munchausen's syndrome, and I gave righteousness to my guilt each night in my insomnia. There are a plethora of options and little to no options all at the same time. I had been scarlet lettered with every scarlet letter I had already branded myself with. I had replayed every moment of my life prior to my pregnancy. Whipping my flesh with every "not of the earth" thing I had put in my mouth. I suffocated myself with every breath of unfiltered air I had taken. I scrubbed my skin until it bled profusely, releasing every drop of perfume and/or body lotion I had poisoned myself with. I killed myself over and over again for everything I had done to my body that inadvertently began to kill her. The irony that solidified my every attempt at suicide was that I was pumping her full of poison, killing her in attempts to save her.

I held the knife to my own throat, beckoning rabbit holes. Those black caves in our brain we avoid like a car swerving away from potholes. Just one small tap on the front tire could be the push that is only followed by an endless spiral. Despite how good of a driver, sometimes the fall is inevitable. Each dirt pebble on its own trip down pushed by a memory from this last year. The waterfall of dust that pours with it is the overwhelming guilt I'm reliving in these days leading up to diagnosis day. There was a muzzle pulled too tight around my jaw and the louder I screamed, the more their heads turn away. With their chin to their chest, they acted as if I weren't even speaking, on mute. It was fuel to my fire, far exceeding its maximum potential. The tsunami hit and blindsided me while riding a longboard with a glass of lemonade adorned with an umbrella. There were flashbacks of this last year and the days in our before. It was like an unedited movie on repeat, with the scenes playing out of order. I still had a constant fear of the night and it was impossible to think beyond tomorrow. I walked this tightrope in stilettos with a weighted vest front and back. There was a faint line between hope and fear every single day. Sometimes my toes would grip the rope. I was able to keep my eyes forward with my belly button tucked to meet my spine, posture strong. I was split second confident that I could see to the other side. The very next step, my foot was too flat and my gaze was lost, hollowed posture. The demons below me, beside me and above, were like a pack of tiger sharks circling chum. The hole swallowed me in one swift swig, while the opening locked and sealed. I know Heaven is home and our forever in the clouds. But I selfishly wanted us to live in the temporary, for just a little while longer. There was not a place in existence where I could live without her next to me. There is no me without her. The crazy was seeping in and there is no sanity in my alive. The tightrope had become the physical vision of my failed attempts at survival. My floating body flailed in the darkness, symbolizing the death of my sane. I was a lost soul, trapped in the in-between. I was attempting to swerve, avoiding the potholes. But sometimes, even savvy drivers can't avoid the crash.

The collision was up ahead and I couldn't see it through my own fog, but I could hear it. Our attempt at keeping her alive was fueling her little body with chemotherapy, so off to clinic we went. She received methotrexate in clinic where I also brought up her leg issues. After an assessment, it was determined that she could possibly be suffering from chemo-induced neuropathy. Dakota was an infant and wasn't able to explain to us what she was feeling so we were constantly throwing paper into the wind when a new symptom arose. There was no treatment for her neuropathy in her treatment for her cancer. The hope was that it would subside once the chemotherapy left her body after treatment. We headed home where I would begin giving her chemotherapy every single day for the rest of the month. This is where the protocol began to change. Up to this point, more often than not, we were in the hospital for treatment. We were slowly turning the tide, as the plan was to continue on with treatment from mostly outside of the hospital. This came with smiles lathered in fear. The hospital had become our safe haven. Although we loathed being there, it had become one of the only places we felt safe. It was the safest place for her in that everyone she needed to keep her alive was there. We had grown accustomed to being with these angels for weeks on end. Even when we went home on vacation, we were still seeing them once a week. The longest time away from them up this point was a two-week span, which felt like years. In those two weeks that felt like an eternity, we choked down our first few rounds of anxiety and PTSD. We had little to no control over most of what was happening in our lives. Being in their presence made us feel as if there was some control, even in the murkiest water.

We had been swimming in these unclear waters for eight months. We watched their every move as they poured poison into our baby's veins. Much of the time, they were suited up in what I can only describe as a thinner version of hazmat suits. Sometimes they wore goggles and they always wore gloves. It wasn't until a few months in that I realized the danger they were putting themselves in constantly, just by being around Dakota. They were pumping what is quite literally poison into her. Therefore, poison was going to seep out of her. Often, she had this smell. The baby smell had died long ago. I would rub my nose into her skin and the hairs inside my nostrils would twitch. She smelled like a laboratory full of chemicals. I only pulled her in closer and the thought alone made me want to burst into tears. The chemo was harvested deep inside her pores and it permeated the air around her. Like the fumes swirling around the poison metal barrel with the big yellow sign adored with a black skull, I gave it a hug. What goes in must come out. I lost count how many times I forgot to put gloves on when I changed her. She was a baby and it was second nature to me to just get in there and clean her up. That couldn't be done with Dakota. The things that were coming out of her were toxic and considered dangerous. She was just this tiny little baby, but her diapers were lethal and not in an amusing way.

Nothing about any of this was funny. I was gearing up to give her poison daily at home. There were these crates that were gifted to me at my baby shower. She was still growing inside me and no one could see the tsunami that was less than a few feet away. The crates were white with blue anchors and her name beautifully written. In her nursey, they held her stuffed animals, crosses and sweet nothings that now were everything. They now held medicated wipes, alcohol wipes, skin prep wipes, syringes, magic mouth wash sponges, nebulizers, calmoseptine, stoma powder, antibacterial bath wipes, oxcycodone, Zofran, chemotherapy and a plethora of other medical necessities. Those crates that were intended as a gift of hope were now my nemeses. I would have to adorn myself in gloves and be sure all objects were clear out of the way in case of splashing when preparing to give her chemo. There were waves of grief that would wash over me, picking at my soul like an ice pick in these moments. Something about having to protect myself from what I was injecting into my infant daughter made my soul howl on its way to its death. I would bite down hard, crunching my teeth to keep the swells from pouring out of my eyes. I had to be insanely precise to fill the exact line despite knowing some would be lost at the top. I am not ashamed to admit, I watched a few videos on filling syringes as I had no other option but than to ace this every single time. This liquid death in this plastic syringe was the only Hail Mary we had at keeping her alive. But I had to wear gloves and be sure not to let it touch my skin as the chemo itself could give me cancer. You have my permission to shake your head. It's beyond an oxymoron. The kicker was that despite the fact that I hated every bit of what we had to do, I wanted to be sure she took in every last drop as I was fearful that if she didn't, her cancer would throw a raging party. It was a sick, twisted and vile club we were in. The noise was deafening and every touch felt like that one pill of ecstasy that would tip over into overdose. We were constantly in a drunken stupor, searching for the exit sign, but there was no escape.

There was no way out, but what we thought was the worst year of our lives was coming to an end. It was New Year's Eve and I was drowning in emotion. I couldn't help but reminisce about how the year began, the events that came as Spring arrived, the crash into the ground with no pause, to today. This year had started with me taking pictures of her in the wee hours of the morning while I pumped and got ready for work. I had thrown myself into giving her a beautiful dedication to God on March 24, not knowing that one month later, to the date, the devil would come for her. I incessantly went back to April 24, assessing every sign I missed. I could still hear my shoes scraping the parking lot of the ER on our way in that unbeknownst to us, was no way out. The ring from the words, "She could die," had never left my ears. His sunken eyes when he said, "She turned purple from the waist up," was still piercing my chest. The weight of her little body in my arms not breathing, is a weight I hadn't yet put down. But carrying her into her first birthday party carried me through. Running my fingers over her chest, there were two things keeping her alive beneath my graze: her port and her heart. We saw her shiny outshine Christmas lights, and my goodness what a sight it was. This year was nothing like we could've ever imagined. It was the year of our death. There were countless casualties. We were not at all who we were in the beginning of the year. We were strangers to ourselves, born in blood. We had endured a never-ending darkness, but we witnessed a blinding light. We had lost almost everything, including ourselves, but she was still here.

$\mathcal{T}$he new year brought a new phase in our new normal. We were at home more often than not, only going to clinic once a month outside of hiccups. It was an adjustment, to say the least, as we had only begun to somewhat gain our bearings in the previous phase. We were outside of the hospital, but the beeping of the machines was still ringing in our ears. Our insomnia was ever present as we had become so accustomed to waking on the hour, every hour. It was in these days, when on paper, things should have eased. But the manifestation of emotions and the mental anguish force the body to shut down in ways that leave little to no control. I started experiencing weight loss, stomach pain, incessant headaches and episodes of loss of breath, like an elephant was sleeping on my chest. My husband had started experiencing periods of brain fog, memory difficulties and struggled with the ability to focus for extended periods of time. Paying myself any attention felt self-serving to me, so I shoved my symptoms down and carried on. My husband attempted to find answers, but on paper, he was a normal human being under stress. I don't know that there is a treatment in the world for smiling hard through gritted teeth, pretending as if your world isn't on fire while your child fights to live. My husband would wake every day from minimal sleep, dress himself in a manner that didn't project our child's battle, and present himself outside of our world as if he weren't a dying man oblivious to his own death. He was doing things I could not do, as I was doing things he could not do.

I could not go out there, into the world, pretending our world wasn't being engulfed by the flames of hell. I could not leave Dakota as her not being in my line of vision gave me visions of living without her. He could not endure her pain as he was unable to fix it and by nature, that is what he does. He could not hold her down, listen to her screams or witness her pain, as it constantly reminded him of how he felt he had failed her. We both assumed our roles by assuming our roles. There was not much discussion. We both understood the necessities without words. He knew I wouldn't leave her as I knew he couldn't fix this, but he would kill himself trying as I would kill myself in attempts to keep her alive. The world didn't stop when ours stopped. Bills still had to be paid and the holes in our life rafts needed patching. His body was worn and his mind was beyond tired, but he was going to the ends of the earth to keep us afloat. I had lost count at the number of times I had died at this point, but by the skin of my teeth, I learned to live in the midst of dying.

We were surrounded by the breath of death, always wondering if we were next. In between our watching the sand pour through the glass tunnel, we threw glitter at the wall and created our own sunshine. At home, I would sing songs and whisper, "I'm sorries," while pushing chemo down her throat. In my undertow of guilt, I would dance while baking and cry hard at the sound of her laugh. That truly was my medicine. In the night, I lived solely on her breaths and clung to the physical presence of her body to keep myself alive. On the eve of clinic nights, I would climb inside myself like a turtle deep inside his shell. I had to shut myself off to others around me in order to prepare for whatever wave was already on its way. I would pack a duffle bag of a week's worth of clothes, just in case we wouldn't be coming home. That in tow with our always packed "go bag," ready for the moments that spared no time for packing. It was a suffocating feeling, packing for the unknown and preparing to be swallowed whole by your worst fears. I would quietly make comfort food in a borrowed kitchen, attempting to fill endless pits that could not be filled. It was always a last supper of sorts as we never knew if we would return or not. We had known all too well at this point what it was like to leave and never return. Therefore, we had become professionals at goodbyes and desensitized to hellos.

God knew we needed hellos and he placed them in the most unexpected places. Driving to clinic was gut-wrenching as I watched everything we knew all too well fade behind us. I had no idea what was ahead of us, but nonetheless, I drove towards our unknown. Thankfully, she would fall asleep on the car ride so I would grant grace while I lost myself in my tears. I needed the release, as pulling into the children's infusion center parking lot required war paint. With black lines drawn under my eyes and her sewn in at my hip, we entered the ring, not knowing how many rounds we would be required to stand and fight. Just as we had begun to lose our grip due to the sweat from blood pressures, a hello arrived. It came in the form of a woman whose husband and sister-in-law I had worked closely with in my former life. She sat with me in my defeat and enticed Dakota with a purple egg shaker to distract her from the boo boos. We were encased in our ice box room, but we could hear the warmth outside of our door. There were sounds of fun, music, tapping feet and laughter. We cautiously opened the door to our igloo and a wave like a blanket pulled us in. Another warrior, near and dear to our hearts, was dancing as only she can, lighting up a room like fireworks to a night sky. Other warriors were drawn to her light and before we could blink, a dance party with chemo poles and tubes had consumed a space that held no space. Dakota was the youngest in the room with her eyes wide at the sight. But not before long, she made her way over to the circle of strength and joined in on the magic.

It was better than unicorns swimming in the skies with mermaid tails, catching rainbow marshmallows and playing harps on the corners of stars. We were in a place that would make a dungeon created for evil resemble a five-star resort serving umbrella drinks. Children were bald and frail, with poison flowing down bloody rivers, hoping to make it through the night to see tomorrow. Yet, warriors were building mountains of strength brick by brick by creating a normal in their disgustingly not normal. It was in moments like these when I learned how to stay alive despite our deaths. There is no brighter light than that of children shining in spite of their dark. In these spaces that held no space, God squeezed in hellos, not out of human desire, but from the necessity of the soul. With our hearts more than content, she was well enough to exit the sunshine after the storm. We said goodbye to our new hellos that were, from this day on, our forever. We drove back to our in-between with heavy eyelids, but lifted spirits. We had been struggling to remain alive while warding off death mentally, emotionally and physically. Our breath was revived by those who were too, living in the midst of battling death. There is nothing more powerful than that of a willed soul. Not even the devil himself in the form of liquid poison or abnormal cells known as cancer stood a chance against the light of child warriors.

191

The light of these warriors brought sunshine to the darkest of days. Even on snowy days at home, Dakota's smile gave warmth to the bitterness outside. Inside, she entertained the room by handing out heart attacks as she was climbing everything in sight. Not being tied to a pole or being bound by the tubes in her chest, opened the door wide to freedom. She was pushing her tiny self to attain heights independently and laughing at the rocking of the furniture's legs beneath her. I had some toddler gymnastics mats delivered to safely encourage her need for mobility. The gymnast inside of me was doing leaps watching her log roll. The cancer mom I had become was cringing each time she chose to dive or jump instead of cautiously depart. Her laugh was intoxicating as it almost mocked the height of the mats themselves. She was far too prepared for challenges and never once winced at the possible fall. Instead, she smiled out of the corner of her mouth and went toward her challenges with vengeance. No matter how many times she fell, she got back up one more time, every single time. Her sitting atop of those mats was like a gold medalist on the platform. She was winning her fight by refusing to accept defeat from her battle.

In the morning, she would bite back at my attempts to get her to swallow down her chemo. But her rejection of defeat came in many forms throughout the day. She would play in the snow for brief periods of time. She was enthralled by its glittering beauty, but not at all a fan of its bluster. She much preferred watching it glisten from behind the window pane. Especially when the smell of chocolate cookies permeated the house. She was in love with the mess of baking and even more so drunk with the taste of sweets. She adored a good cuddle session, wrapped three times in a warm fuzzy blanket. She fought medications hard, both morning and night. Something about the night time dose upset her stomach far more so than in the morning, causing vomiting. Her projectile episodes upset her beyond being consoled and often bled into bedtime. This would warrant a passing of her tiny squirming body from one person to the next. Her head was either on a left shoulder or listening to the beat of a heart inside a trusted body's chest. Her thumb was fully inserted, holding back some of the depths of her cries. *Moana* or her Pop Pop's music would be playing in the background in hopes of bringing her storm to a settle. Sometimes all of our tactics would work for brief periods, but never for a full night's sleep. She was still up often throughout the night. At times, she was still howling at the moon. Other times, she just wanted to be up in someone's arms. Her nights were often more restless than her days, but despite her tired, she forged on.

She was full steam ahead in no way any one-year-old should have to be, but she did so anyway. We were still working on pottying to decrease the amount of chemo damage to her most gentle areas. I caught much backlash as my introducing the potty came off forceful. I can't say or not say that I would have waited or done exactly the same schedule if our situation had been different. But the truth was, I was simply doing what any mother would do for her child, which was to decrease any amount of pain that her child may endure. I had seen Dakota's area look as if it had been held to flames for hours on end. I had seen blood and blisters in places that should never exist. I had scorned images in my head that will haunt me for the rest of my days. I was doing the best I could in the lose/lose situation I was in, to keep my baby from suffering. I was swinging my bat at the same scrutiny I was receiving for pushing her daily in academics to decrease the impact of chemo brain. Again, I can't say for sure if my parenting would have been any different outside of our situation. But upon being informed of all of the horrific things that could happen to her and/or the things that would debilitate her throughout her life, all while fighting for her life, I had to make incredibly difficult decisions. I chose to give her the best chance at the life she would live for as many days as she would live it. I was not making her sit in a sweat box with rice beneath her bottom. I was taking a few minutes out of our every day to review colors, shapes, letters and to read. I see how that could be considered drastic for a barely one-year-old, but it was not drastic in the hurdles we were facing up ahead. If we made it that far.

We would climb mountains in a little red wagon, but she couldn't be in the sun because of chemo side effects. We placed towels over the sides of the wagon's canopy to decrease the amount of sunlight that may graze her skin. We were throwing glitter at the wall, giving her time outside as any child deserves, but throwing hail Mary's to be sure the outside didn't hurt her. She looked like a princess encased in her carriage except I was the horse. My legs were tired and my lungs had no breath left to give, but her laugh was all the momentum I needed to uphold my endurance. I loathed the way we had to, but I was more than grateful that we got to. I savored the exhausting, but joyous moment as we were headed to clinic in the morning. The unknown was on the horizon and all we had was now.

Every fighter and those who walk beside them, know one thing and one thing only: all there is, is now. After the initial hit of diagnosis, the world splits in two. There is the world you once knew that you will never fully exist in again. There is the world of cancer, fighting, poison, death and destruction that you will never escape. There is you, and you will forever exist somewhere in between, but you will not be alone. The very essence of you becomes something that people outside of the cancer world turn away from. Rightfully so, as it is so grotesque that there are no words. Without whispering a word, they are grateful it's not them, and you wish like hell they could understand your pain, in the same breath you protect them from it. But their shoes are nothing like yours and the paths up ahead are forever diverged. There are people who walk beside you with shoes, worn and tattered, just as yours are. They have holes embedded deep inside them that will never be filled in. Their shoulders carry an unseen amount of weight, but the hunch of their back showcases just how heavy it really is. Their lips force a smile, but you can hear the chattering in their teeth. Their eyes are hollow, cold, bright and shiny all within the same blink. They are the mirror image of you, and without a word spoken, it is understood. No words need to be said because they hear you through closed lips. You are all climbing the same endless hills with no decline, with shackles laced around your ankles and chains buried deep in the earth. All of you exist inside of a bubble birthed in hell stealing glimpses of the butterflies and sunshine out there. There is absolute jealousy, but more so, a gratitude in that, although it would be glorious to slide down those rainbows into a pit of smothered sundaes, we are forever grateful for every day we are gifted in here.

195

On this night before counts and methotrexate, there were multiple fighters just like Dakota, battling demons to have a chance to see tomorrow's light. I walked with them in their grief because I knew their grief. I spoke with them through the darkness of the night as I too, was lost in the unseen awaiting dawn. I held space for them in the space where I could not physically hold them and I held them anyway. To the outsiders, these were self-inflicted wounds and pain at my own hand. But to me, this was the only place outside of her breath that I found my own breath. Hand-in-hand with those just like us felt like the home we didn't have. Standing with fighters who knew our fight chipped away at our alone and cemented dirt beneath our feet that were desperately searching for ground. We were more than alone, but together.

Together, we were gloving up to protect our pores from drinking in the poison we were pumping down our child's throat. We were making 20 different meals a day, and throwing cheese sticks in our fighter's direction in the hopes that something would go down the hatch. We were sledding down hills of ice that held more warmth than what was left of our souls in attempts to give our child the life they so very much deserve. We were analyzing red rashes that caused our hearts to splatter beneath our tattered shoes. All the while, assisting teams of the most intelligent angels in filling our child with toxins in hopes of giving her life. We had one foot in and one foot out. Some days outside of the hospital mixing chocolate pudding with the devil's juice. Other days, we were clawing at hospital walls trying to not let anyone witness the actual kiss of our head on the concrete. We were laughing and crying between the steroid-induced Jekyll and Hyde our child had involuntarily become. Walking around daily half awake as our bodies and our minds had completely quit the idea of sleep. Instead, we held our warrior close as her body melted from the inside out due to the overwhelming number of venoms boiling inside its blood. We found escapes from our insanity in brief periods with hair cuts and all too short visits with those who still looked at us. Our words made their ears bleed as we couldn't help but speak of the horrors of watching our baby release blood curdling screams despite her eyes closed, the very definition of helplessness. Our Bandaids were the videos of our infant walking for the first time despite the death coursing through her veins. Some from the other world still stood with us by choice. Others who were forced into our world, walked with us both in grief and honor.

With our heads hung in fear, yet grateful hearts, we went to clinic for methotrexate and antibodies to assist her immune system. She was not considered neutropenic, but she was right on the cusp, therefore we were to treat her and her environment as such. We were forced to live in a certain manner in hopes of keeping Dakota as well as possible and alive. We, in no way, wanted to push our have to on others and the water was growing murkier by the day. She had little to no appetite and our nights were worsening rather than improving. We had been in treatment just a few months shy of one year up to this point. For more than 90 percent of this last year, we had been in the hospital more than we had not. Our being in the hospital was much less intrusive to others' day-to-day lives as we were not there. When we were outside of the hospital, we still had to maintain our lifestyle of isolation in hopes of keeping Dakota safe. This became problematic in a full house as we could not expect others outside of our world to live as we had to inside of our world. We were blessed to have people in our lives who were willing to turn their lives upside down in order to help us. The lines were blurred in that we had no choice but to live this way. Our way of living that had no choice was negatively affecting the lives of others who still had a choice. Our life was still on pause while other lives were still on play. No one was in the wrong, but nothing was right.

As it was, we were approaching her last full week in clinic, receiving chemotherapy and fluids. These days were open to close, and drained every drop of human we had remaining. The car ride home was almost as horrific as the every 15-minute blood pressures. She screamed through her living nightmare the entire drive. Our minds held no sane thoughts and our bodies had transformed into liquid. We were less than half way through our marathon and closer to death mentally, more so now, than we were just a few months ago, physically. Other babies who were swinging swords beside us were dying.

Choking down our sobs, we forged on with chemo, Neupogen® shots, Bactrim, "methotrexate Mondays" and pulses of dexamethasone. Dakota was transitioning into the maintenance phase of her treatment. This phase consisted of daily chemo morning and night, Bactrim on the weekends to prevent lung infections, methotrexate on Mondays for a little splash of evil, and a five-day pulse of steroids to add a cherry on top. We began this phase on March 2, 2020, and despite its hellish laugh, it gave wind to our wings. In this phase, we were encouraged to begin tasting pieces of normal again. This was a hard pill to swallow as we had completely forgotten what normal was, and we still had whiplash from our new normal. Up to this point since April of the previous year, grass was a danger, the sun was a threat and bodies of water were an absolute no. The only safety we had known was our bubble, and its pop was blowing out our eardrums. Despite the ringing in our ears, we let our sneakers hit the pavement, and we not only walked, we ran. Dakota's feet touched grass for the first time since our before. She saw ducks, dogs that weren't in homes, and she couldn't stop herself from saying, "Oh wow!" She wasn't eating much, but she tasted chocolate ice cream in a cone from the inside of a parlor. She sat in awe of a stream of water from inside in her stroller as I ran to the beat of my feet kissing the pavement. We jumped in puddles and witnessed the stillness of a lake from afar. Our wings were just beginning to stretch and we were preparing to take flight. The devil mocked our fully embraced drops of freedom swimming on our lips as he kissed the world with a pandemic.

On March 11, 2020, the world was blanketed with a global virus. No one had answers and everyone was right in their wrong. The arrow on the wheel was spinning as we all waited anxiously for direction. There was no book on how to navigate a pandemic, let alone how to keep a child battling cancer alive during a pandemic, but here we were. Everyone was making valiant efforts to do their best in remaining safe to help keep Dakota as healthy as humanly possible. But despite the world now enduring a pause, life continued on play. We closed our doors just as quickly as we had opened them. We were veterans as we had already been living a life of isolation for the last 11 months. With the help of disinfectant wipes and a multitude of masks, we encased ourselves more deeply in individualized bubbles, in hopes of keeping Dakota alive. Despite holding our breath and warding off physical touch, we were barely treading water in our ocean of panic. We had come so far in our forever journey and we had just a little over one year left, living in survival mode and hoping to see tomorrow. A fury had engulfed us as we couldn't fathom escaping death this many times to be possibly taken out by a virus. Everyone was angry and everyone's anger was more than validated. The world outside was dark and its storm was beginning to seep through the cracks at the bottom of our doors. There was no touch as touch had become lethal. There was no listening as the noise had become deafening. There was nothing to do in the overwhelming to dos. So, I reached through the dark and whispered, "I see you."

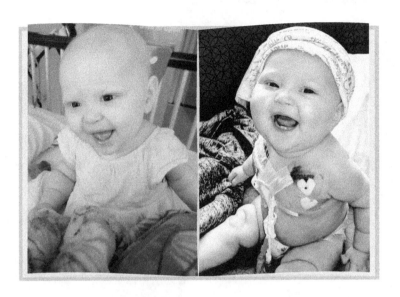

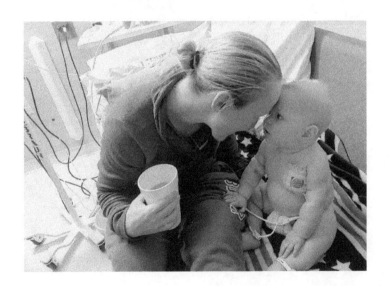

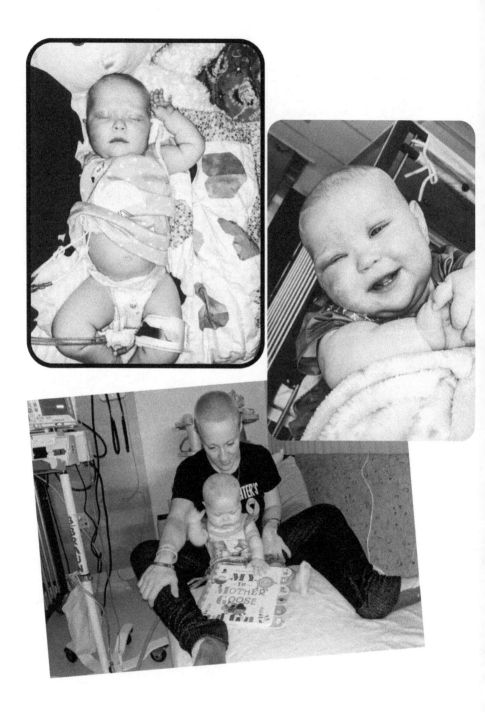

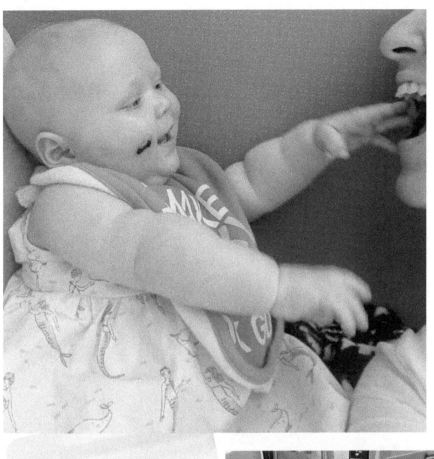
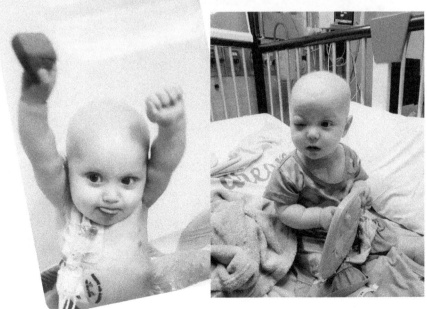

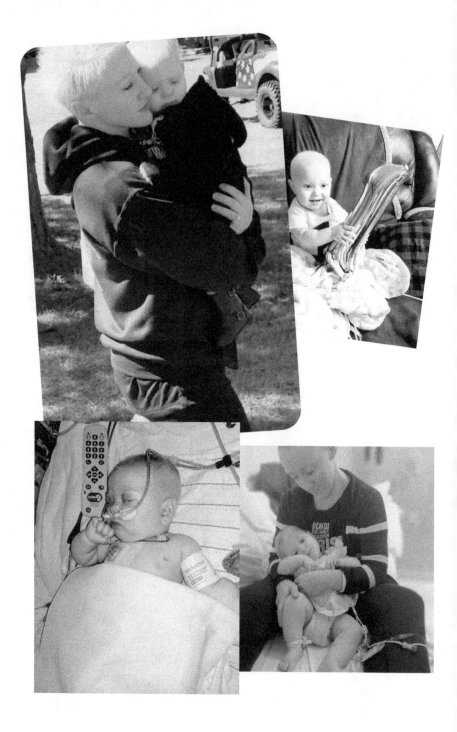

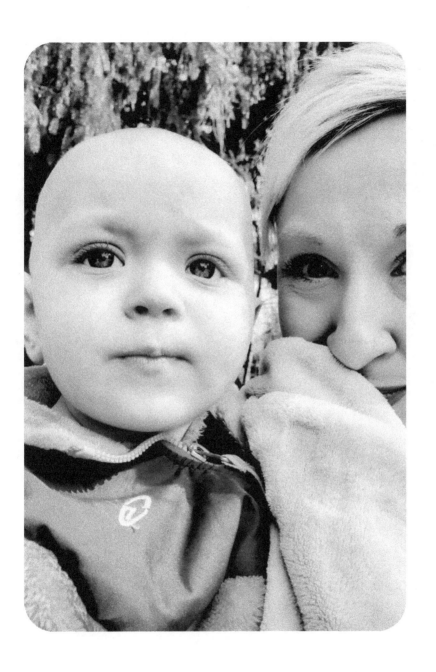

ABOUT THE AUTHOR

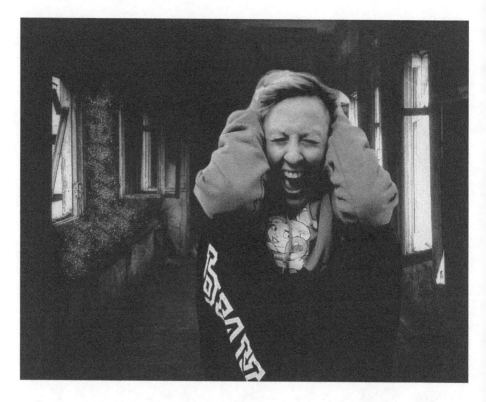

Shari Ann Almeida lives with her husband and four-year-old daughter, Dakota Ann, in North Carolina. Her work with Warrior Moms United by Pediatric Cancer (and now Warrior Dads) continues out of its base in Lehigh Valley Pennsylvania.

She also assists with other local chapters of Warrior Moms United by Pediatric Cancer in different states. If you or someone you know is a cancer mom in search of community, please contact Shari Ann for assistance.

To contact her, send a message through Facebook Messenger @Shari Ann Almeida.

Look for more of her work coming soon as the story continues.

CPSIA information can be obtained
at www.ICGtesting.com
Printed in the USA
BVHW030004230123
656884BV00002B/10

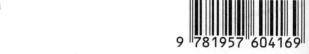